SKILLED AND VOCATIONAL TRADES

BECOME A
HOME
HEALTH AIDE

by Philip Wolny

BrightPoint Press

San Diego, CA

BrightPoint Press

© 2024 BrightPoint Press
an imprint of ReferencePoint Press, Inc.
Printed in the United States

For more information, contact:
BrightPoint Press
PO Box 27779
San Diego, CA 92198
www.BrightPointPress.com

ALL RIGHTS RESERVED.

No part of this work covered by the copyright hereon may be reproduced or used in any form or by any means—graphic, electronic, or mechanical, including photocopying, recording, taping, web distribution, or information storage retrieval systems—without the written permission of the publisher.

LIBRARY OF CONGRESS CATALOGING-IN-PUBLICATION DATA

Names: Wolny, Philip, author.
Title: Become a home health aide / by Philip Wolny.
Description: San Diego, CA: BrightPoint Press, [2024] | Series: Skilled and vocational trades | Includes bibliographical references and index. | Audience: Ages 13 | Audience: Grades 7-9
Identifiers: LCCN 2023000093 (print) | LCCN 2023000094 (eBook) | ISBN 9781678206840 (hardcover) | ISBN 9781678206857 (eBook)
Subjects: LCSH: Home health aides--United States--Juvenile literature. | Home care services--Vocational guidance--United States--Juvenile literature.
Classification: LCC RA645.35 .W65 2024 (print) | LCC RA645.35 (eBook) | DDC 362.14023--dc23/eng/20230420
LC record available at https://lccn.loc.gov/2023000093
LC eBook record available at https://lccn.loc.gov/2023000094

CONTENTS

AT A GLANCE	4
INTRODUCTION	6
THE FRONT LINE OF CAREGIVING	
CHAPTER ONE	12
WHAT DOES A HOME HEALTH AIDE DO?	
CHAPTER TWO	26
WHAT TRAINING DO HOME HEALTH AIDES NEED?	
CHAPTER THREE	44
WHAT IS LIFE LIKE AS A HOME HEALTH AIDE?	
CHAPTER FOUR	60
WHAT IS THE FUTURE FOR HOME HEALTH AIDES?	
Glossary	74
Source Notes	75
For Further Research	76
Index	78
Image Credits	79
About the Author	80

AT A GLANCE

- Home health aides are an important part of the nation's health care system. They look out for the well-being of many sick, elderly, and disabled people living at home.

- Home health aides have many jobs. Their main responsibilities are helping their patients with bathing, feeding, cleaning, exercise, errands, and other tasks.

- Home health aides are either trained on the job or do training courses to meet the requirements for working in people's homes.

- Training programs and courses at places such as vocational schools and community colleges teach health aides the basics of taking care of patients.

- Being a home health aide is a tough job, both mentally and physically. Aides must be physically strong and able to deal with stress.

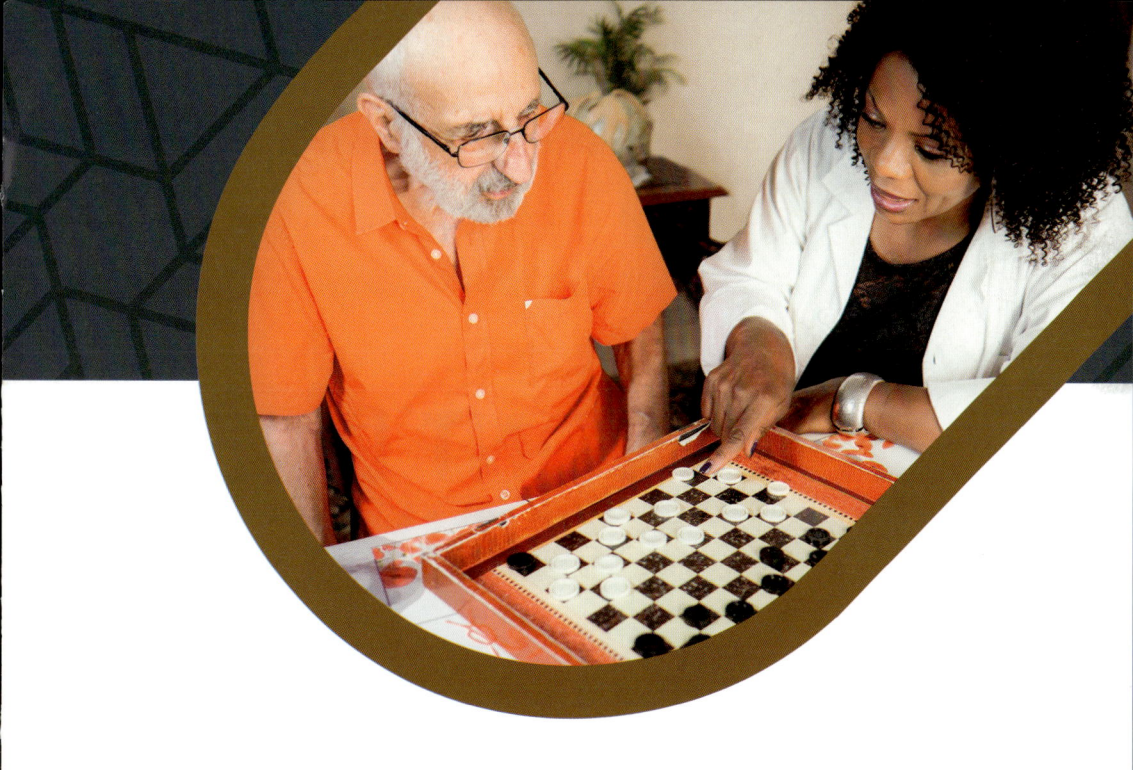

- Caring for patients can be a messy and unpleasant experience. Health aides must keep themselves and their patients safe.

- The need for health aides is expected to grow over the next decade. There is a current shortage of health aides for those who need them.

- Improving the pay, working conditions, and status of health aides will help employers hire the help that millions of patients need. New laws and government funding could help improve the state of home care in the future.

INTRODUCTION

THE FRONT LINE OF CAREGIVING

On an early morning in Stamford, Connecticut, seventy-seven-year-old Bob Dettmer banged on a bedroom door. He was in his own house. But he was yelling that he wanted to go home.

It was a common experience for Marjorie Salmon. She was not his wife or relative. She wasn't a family member or even a

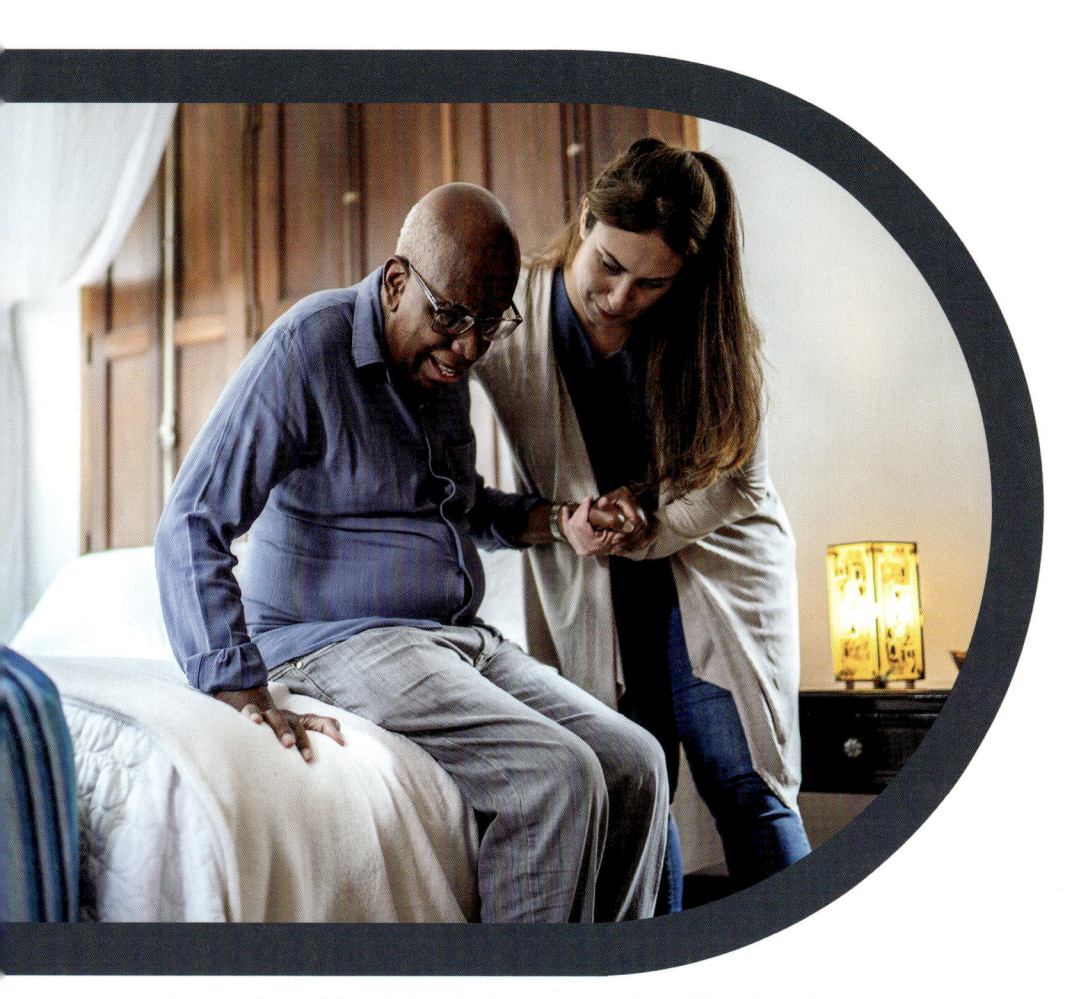

Home health aides take care of patients who cannot take care of themselves.

friend. She had been Dettmer's home health aide for a few months. Dettmer had Parkinson's disease. That made it hard for him to move around. He also had

Alzheimer's disease. It made him forget many things. It could also make him confused, scared, and even angry. That was why he was knocking loudly on her bedroom door at 4:00 a.m.

Salmon was a live-in health aide. While taking care of Dettmer, she lived at his home full time. She worked about 26 or 27 days out of the month. Dettmer's family paid her $160 per day. She cooked and cleaned. She often changed Dettmer's adult diaper. She also did dozens of other tasks. A *New York Times* article compared Salmon's job to being a babysitter, nurse,

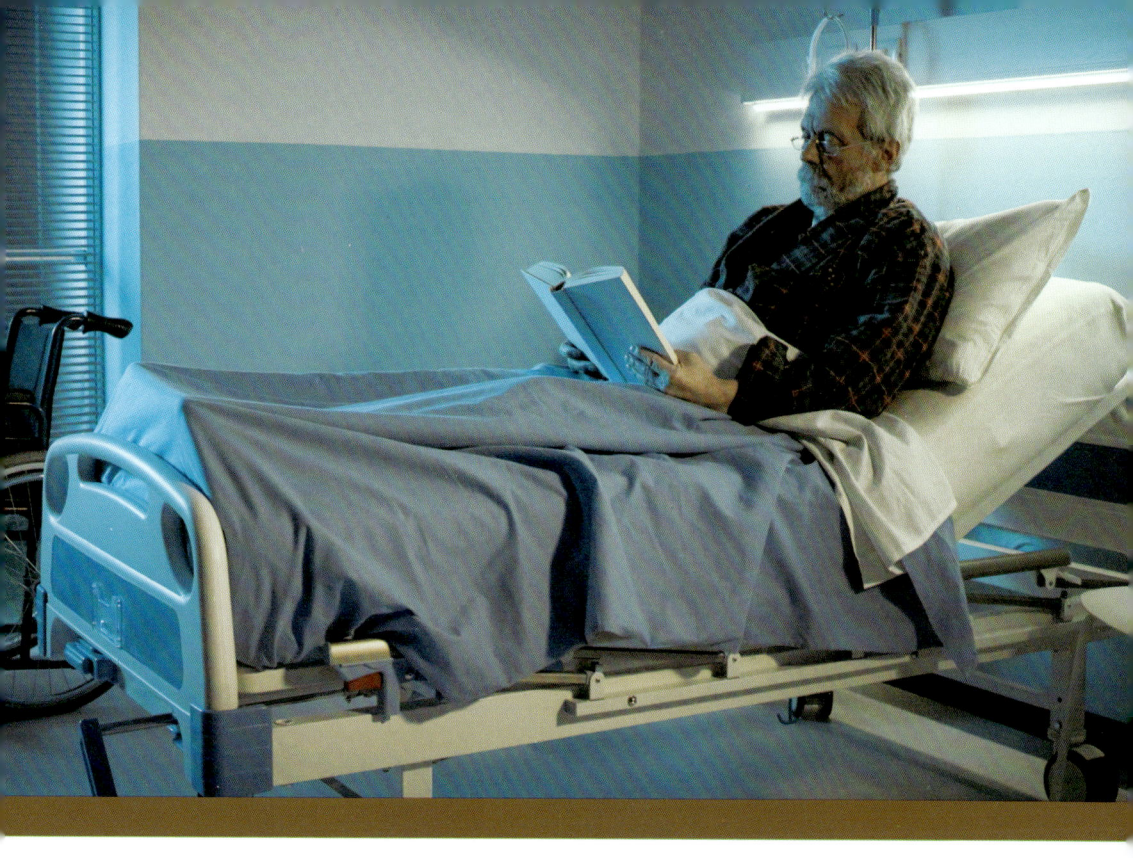

For many patients, receiving care at home is much better than receiving care in a hospital.

therapist, parent, and housekeeper, all at the same time.

Being a home health aide can be rewarding. It can also be stressful and tiring. Home health aides are a huge part of the health care profession. Without them,

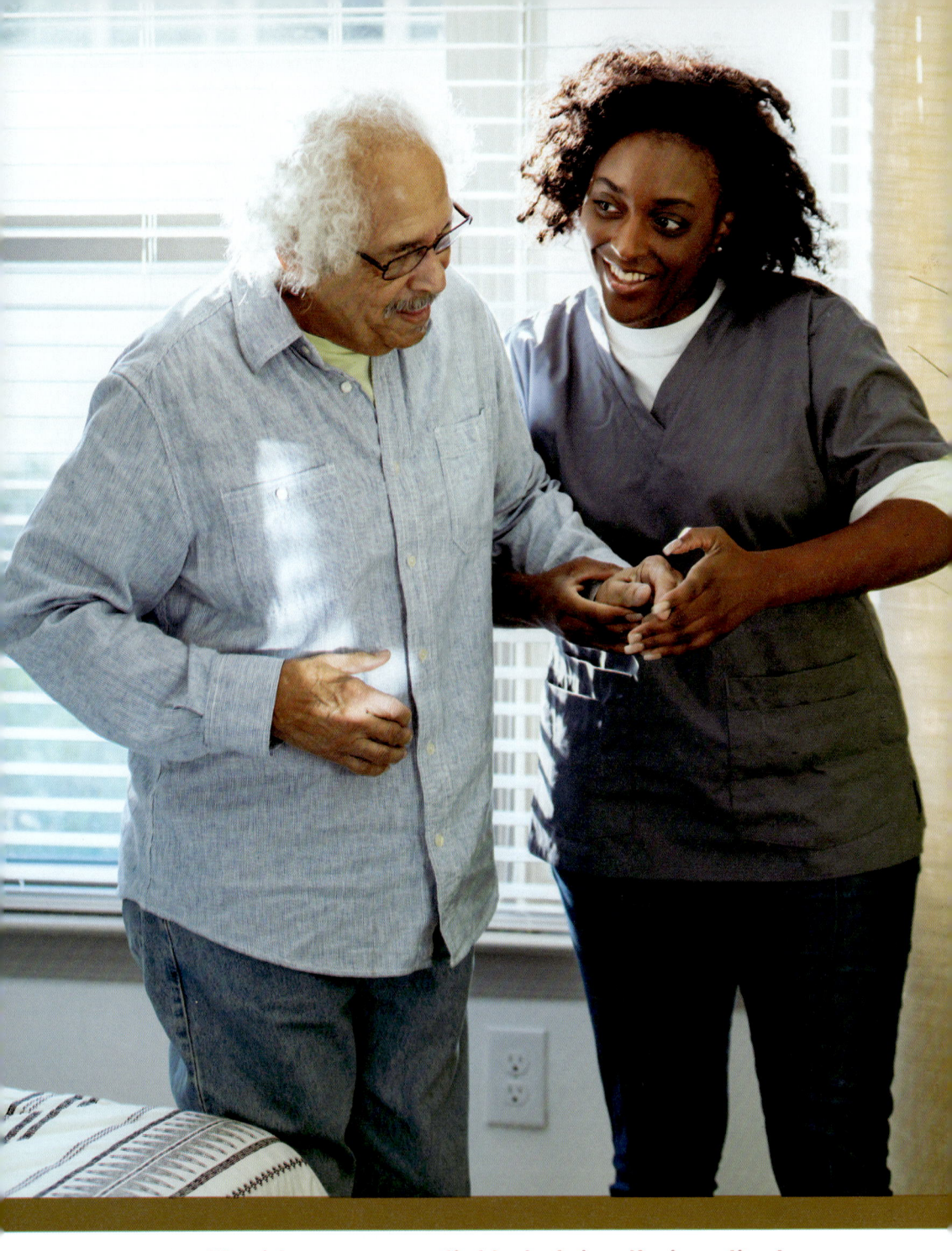

Health aides are essential to helping their patients maintain independence in their own homes.

millions of patients would have to receive care in nursing homes or hospitals.

Health aides are committed caregivers. They work with some of the most **vulnerable** people in society. Being a health aide requires physical and mental strength. It is a great job for someone who cares about people. Health aides must think on their feet. They must deal with situations that many other people do not want to handle. The need for more home health aides is expected to grow in the future.

CHAPTER ONE

WHAT DOES A HOME HEALTH AIDE DO?

When people hear the phrase *health care*, they may think of hospitals, clinics, doctors, and nurses. But there are many lesser-known health care workers who are just as important. Millions of patients depend on them. These workers are known as home health aides.

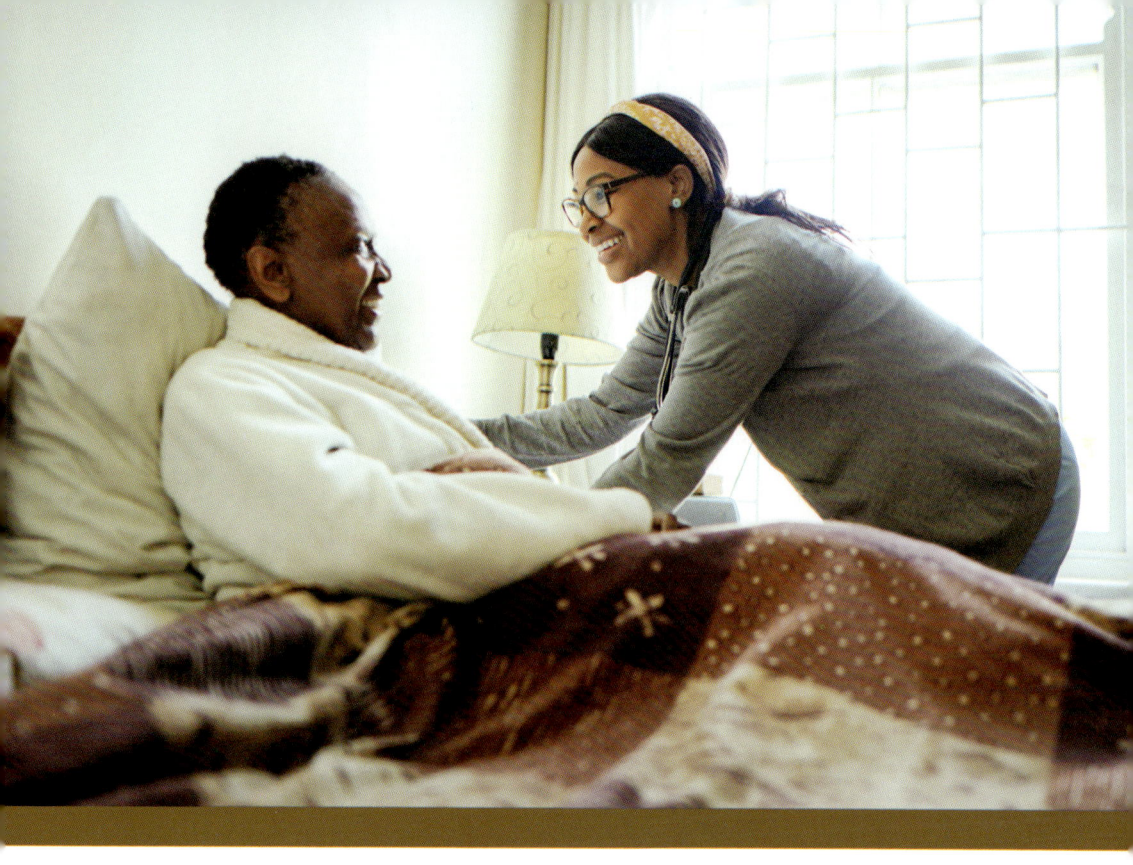

Home health aides are very important in the health care industry.

Many Americans with medical issues need help to get through their days. This includes seniors. It also includes people living with major disabilities or health issues. People who are recovering from injuries might need help. Some needs are temporary. Others involve long-term care. Health aides help address all of these needs.

The home care industry grew quickly over the last few decades. Medicine and technology have helped older Americans live longer. However, many do not want to go to nursing or retirement homes. Home health aides can help people stay in their own homes.

HOME IS WHERE THE HELP IS

Nurses and doctors usually work in hospitals. Home health aides work in the private homes of patients. The aides'

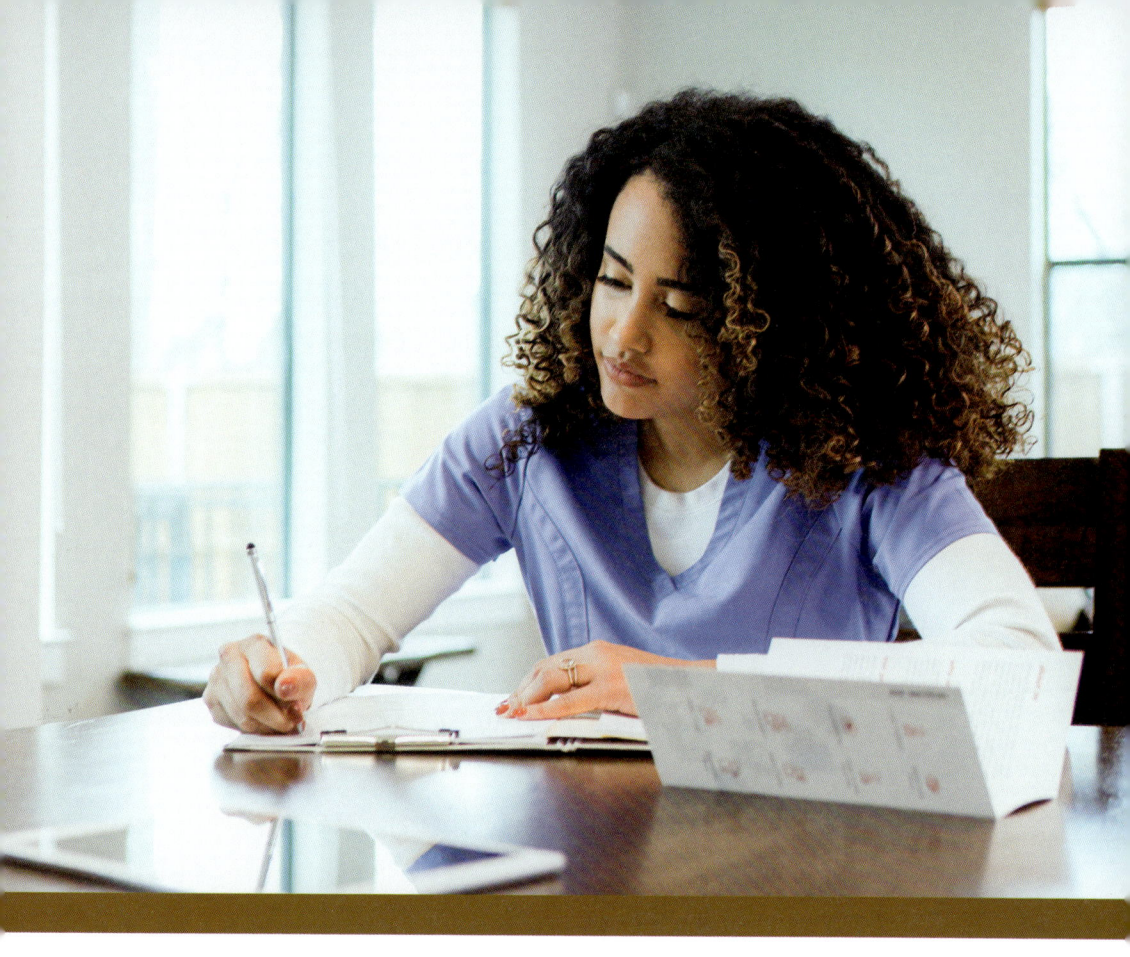

For home health aides who visit multiple patients per day, it is good to write down records of each patient's medication and condition.

responsibilities can vary depending on their patient. Some patients need more help than others.

Sometimes patients do not have family support. They need overnight help from live-in caregivers. Health aides might live with these patients long term. This is especially true for people with major health issues or disabilities. These aides are always in contact with their patient's doctors.

Most health aides in the United States work for home health agencies. These agencies are often private companies. Some aides work for nonprofit groups. Others are hired directly by local, state, and federal governments. Government programs like Medicare and Medicaid provide care to seniors and those with low incomes.

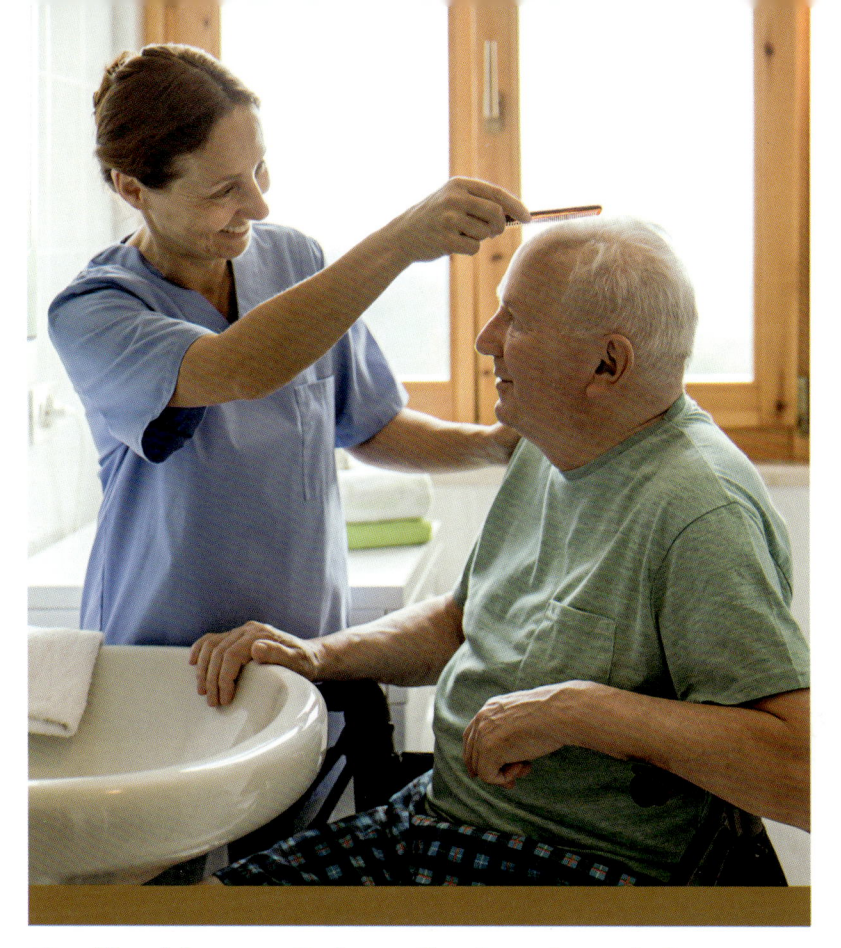

Health aides can help patients get ready in the morning.

THE MANY JOBS OF A HEALTH AIDE

Home health aides must help patients with things they cannot do by themselves. These are often called "Activities of Daily Living," or ADLs for short. ADLs are basic tasks a patient may need help with. This includes tasks like getting to the bathroom. Such patients need help showering, shaving, or bathing. They also need someone to help them get dressed. Other patients may not be able to get in and out of bed. They might need help getting into a wheelchair. A health aide may help with crutches and other **mobility aids**. This ADL can be challenging.

Instrumental ADLs (IADLs) are more complex tasks. IADLs can include light housekeeping, such as cleaning and doing laundry. Aides might shop for and

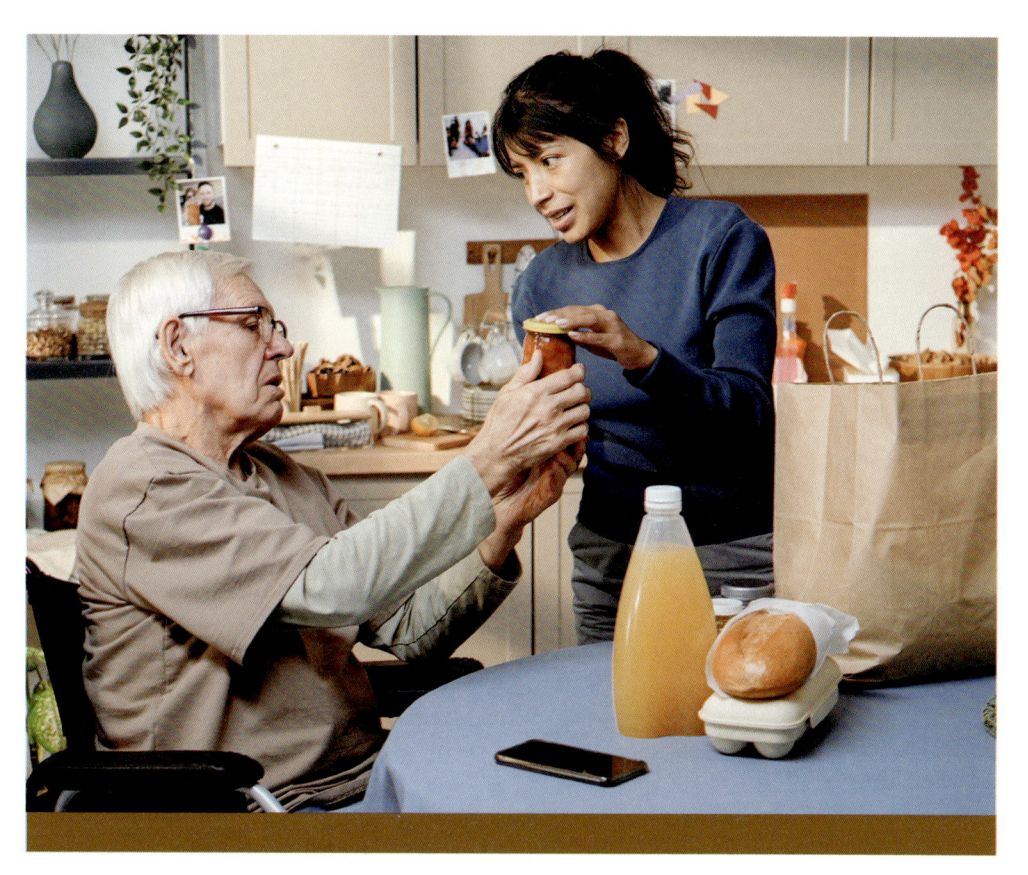

Health aides may help patients with everyday activities like shopping for food.

prepare meals. They will also clean up afterward. Health aides may help patients manage their medications.

Another IADL is helping patients keep appointments. Aides may take patients to hospitals or clinics. Patients might need to go shopping. Aides may take patients to meet friends and family. They might also simply take them out for some fresh air. Deborah O'Bryant told *The Guardian* about her time as a home health aide to a cancer patient. She said, "I had to take her to radiation every day. She could not speak. I learned how to read lips."[1]

Elderly, sick, and disabled people can suffer from being alone. Depression is a common mental illness for them. Aides can help patients reconnect with loved ones and their favorite activities.

Besides these ADLs and IADLs, some patients need physical activity. Exercise can help them recover from surgery or an injury. Moving around often is good for their health. It can positively affect their mental well-being. Health aides may also help with patients' aches and pains. They can

A HUMAN TOUCH

Some patients rarely see friends or family. Others have no one at all. A health aide might be the only person a patient sees. An aide's visit can lift their spirits. Having conversations, playing board games or cards, or simply watching a video together can improve a patient's spirits. It can even improve their health.

massage their patients or help them stretch. Performing some basic motions in bed can help blood flow.

MONITORING MEDICATIONS AND HEALTH

Health aides must make sure patients take their medications. That process can look different depending on the state. Many states do not let aides give medications directly to patients. Instead, health aides can only bring medications to their patients. They also bring items that will help the patient take the medication. This might include water.

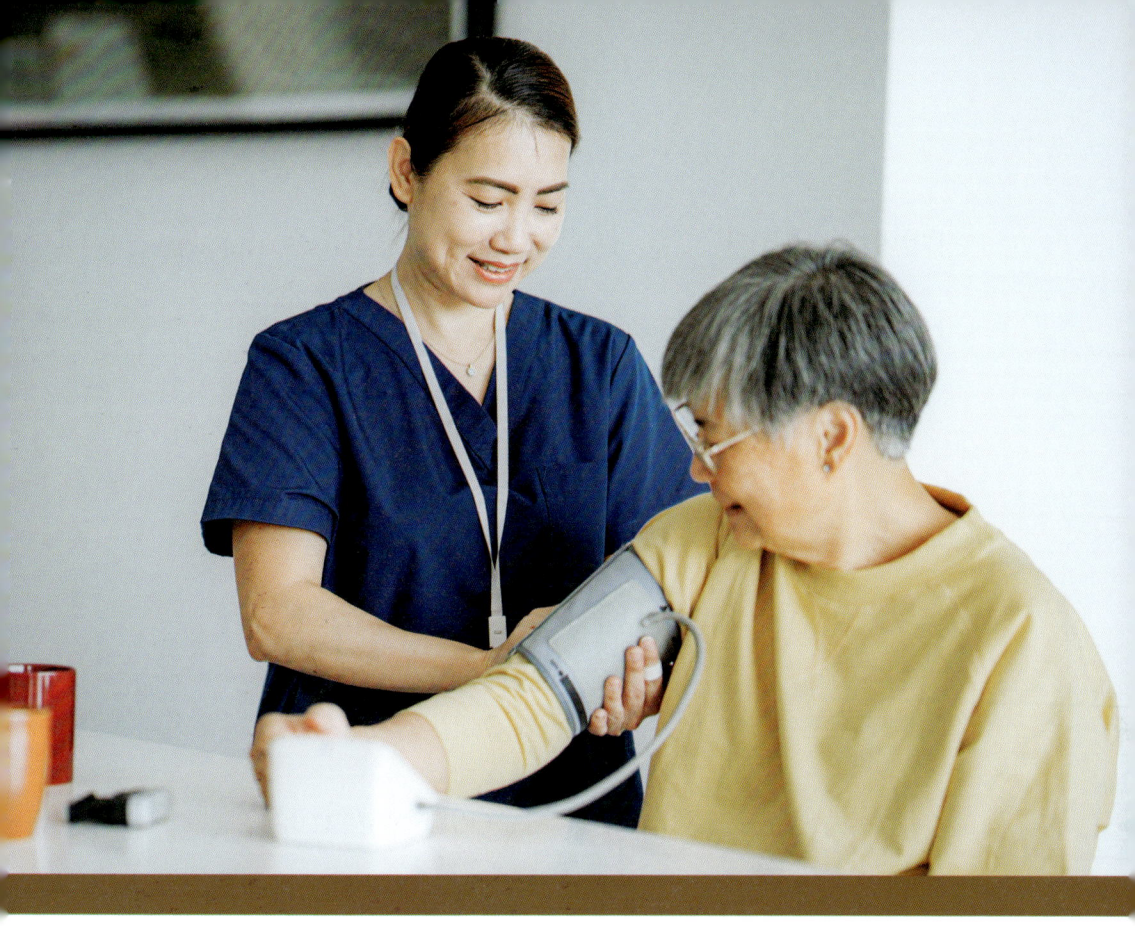

Knowing how to measure blood pressure is an important skill for health aides.

Depending on the state, aides can do other things to monitor a patient's condition. They can check their temperature with a thermometer. They can check a patient's pulse. Aides can also monitor patient breathing. They can measure blood pressure.

Home health aides often do light medical care. In many states, they can change bandages. They might inspect and clean medical equipment.

MANAGING CARE

Health aides are part of a larger team of care professionals. This team can include doctors, nurses, and medical assistants. Aides may also work with other health aides. This is because some patients have more than one health aide taking care of them.

Most of the time, nurses train and supervise aides. Nurses let aides know what medications patients take and when they should take them. Nurses also help health aides plan for any concerns with their patients' health.

PAPERWORK AND COMMUNICATION

Doctors and nurses monitor patient health. Aides provide constant updates about any health issues or changes. Aides need to keep good records. This ensures that doctors and nurses give patients the right medical care. It helps things run smoothly for patients and all their caregivers.

CHAPTER TWO

WHAT TRAINING DO HOME HEALTH AIDES NEED?

Most health aide jobs are **entry-level** positions. In many states, aides only need high school diplomas. Otherwise, they must pass their Graduate Educational Development (GED) test. This is seen as a diploma.

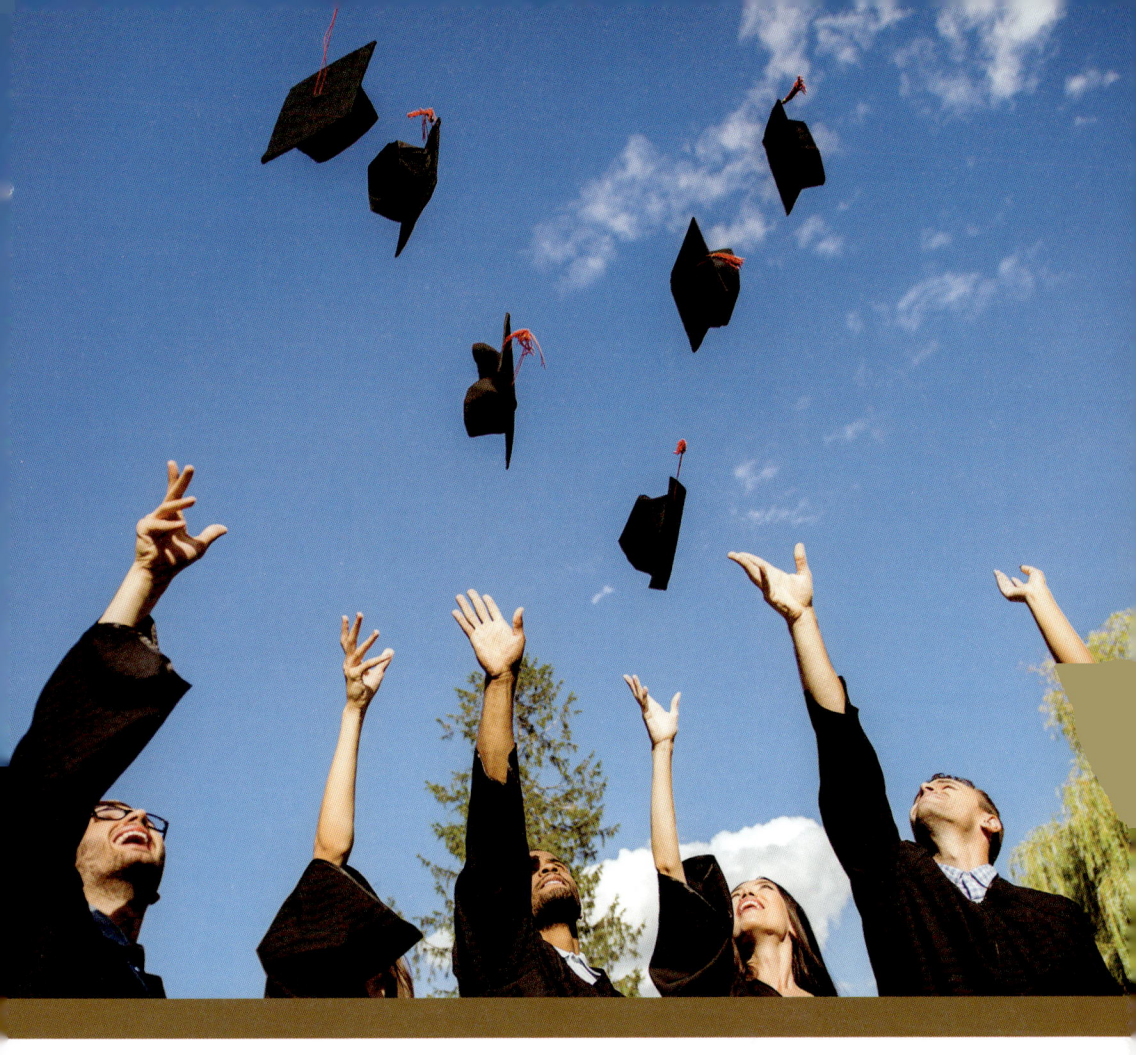

A high school diploma is the basic requirement for most health aide jobs.

Certain states do not require a diploma or GED. Employers can ask applicants to take some tests. Tests might cover reading, math, and English language skills.

However, having a diploma or GED makes getting a job more likely.

Health aides may start their careers with on-the-job training. Going to a vocational school or college is another route. This education can lead to being certified and landing a job. Aides can earn extra certifications. They can also take yearly courses to keep learning.

TRAINING ON THE JOB

Home health agencies train new health aides. Agencies teach aides the basics of housekeeping. Aides must learn food preparation. They need to make healthy

EDUCATION OF HOME CARE WORKERS IN 2020

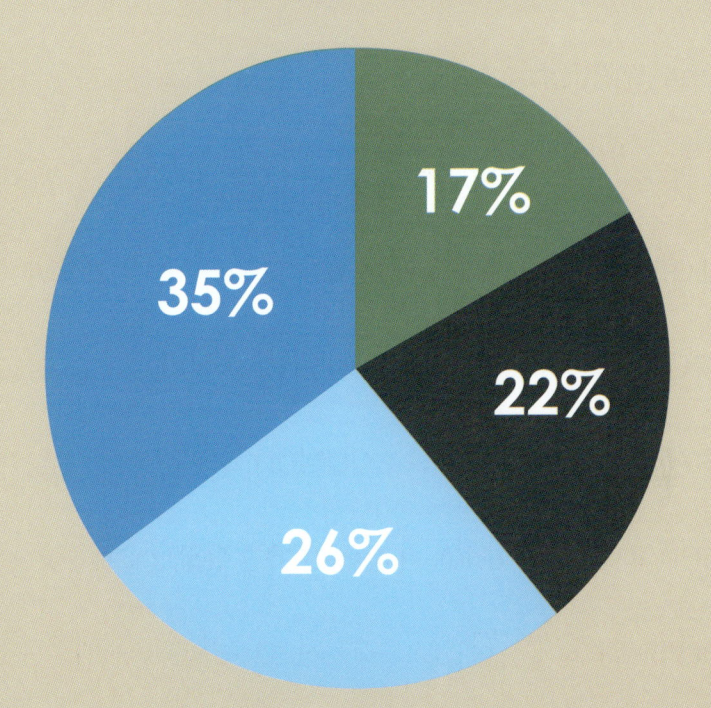

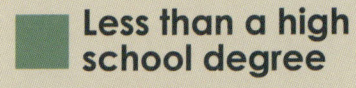

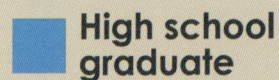

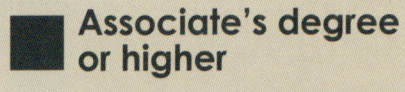

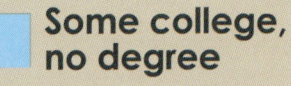

- 17% Less than a high school degree
- 22% Associate's degree or higher
- 26% Some college, no degree
- 35% High school graduate

Source: "U.S. Home Care Workers Key Facts," PHI, 2022. www.phinational.org.

Home care workers include home health aides, nursing assistants, and personal care aides. Many home care workers have graduated high school but have not received any other higher education.

foods for patients with special dietary needs or restrictions.

Aides need to learn basic safety guidelines. They must learn what to do in emergencies. They learn how to bathe and care for patients. In addition, aides must know how to take a patient's temperature and pulse.

GETTING CERTIFIED AND LICENSED

Not all health aide agencies provide training. In some states, agencies only hire aides who are already certified. The National Association for Home Care & Hospice (NAHC) is the biggest national organization that offers certification. Sometimes agencies will only hire those who receive NAHC or equivalent certification.

Some aides work for agencies whose services are paid for by Medicaid or Medicare. Federal law states that these aides must have seventy-five hours

A DRIVER'S LICENSE

Health aides usually need a driver's license. Employers might also need aides to have a clean driving record. Patients need help getting around to appointments and errands. Health aides might also live far from their agency and clients. Public transportation might not be reliable in some areas. It might not be available at all.

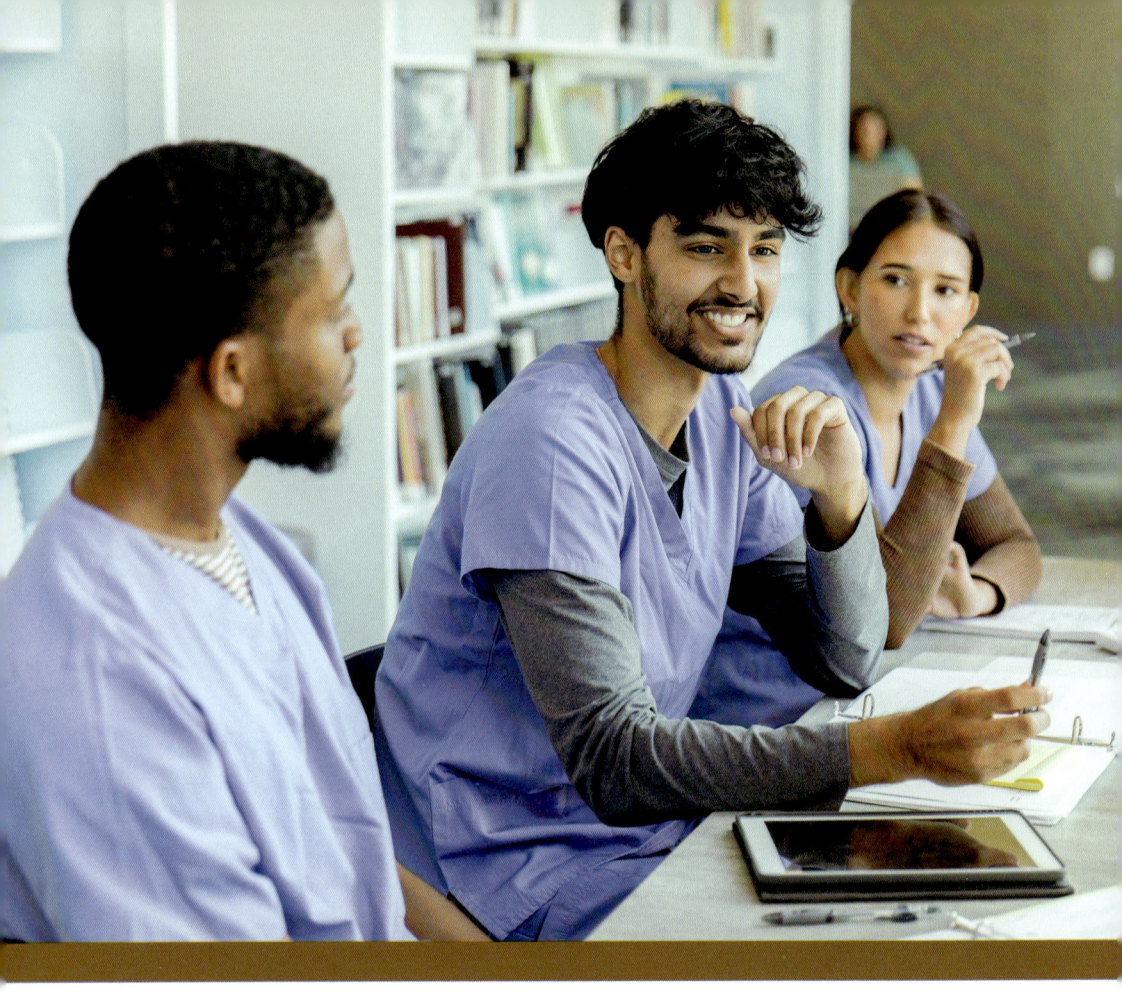

Training programs are usually given in community colleges, nursing schools, adult schools, and health care organizations.

of training. Some states such as Wisconsin require up to 120 hours of training. After training, health aides typically must pass an exam.

Health aides can also take classes at vocational schools that lead to certification. These courses can cost between $300 and $650. More advanced, longer courses that last longer can cost more. Community colleges, junior colleges, and even four-year universities offer courses toward certification.

A health aide might need to contact the NAHC to get certified after taking classes. Some programs might help students with the certification process. Nonprofit organizations and nursing programs may offer coursework that leads to certification.

WHAT HEALTH AIDES LEARN

Most health aide training programs cover similar skills and tasks. California has strict standards for home health aide programs. The total course must be at least 120 hours. Students must spend twenty hours on the medical and social needs of patients. The biggest part of the coursework is on personal care services. This takes about seventy hours.

When students learn about personal care services, they are taught how to help patients with **hygiene** and mobility. Mobility training can include helping patients move

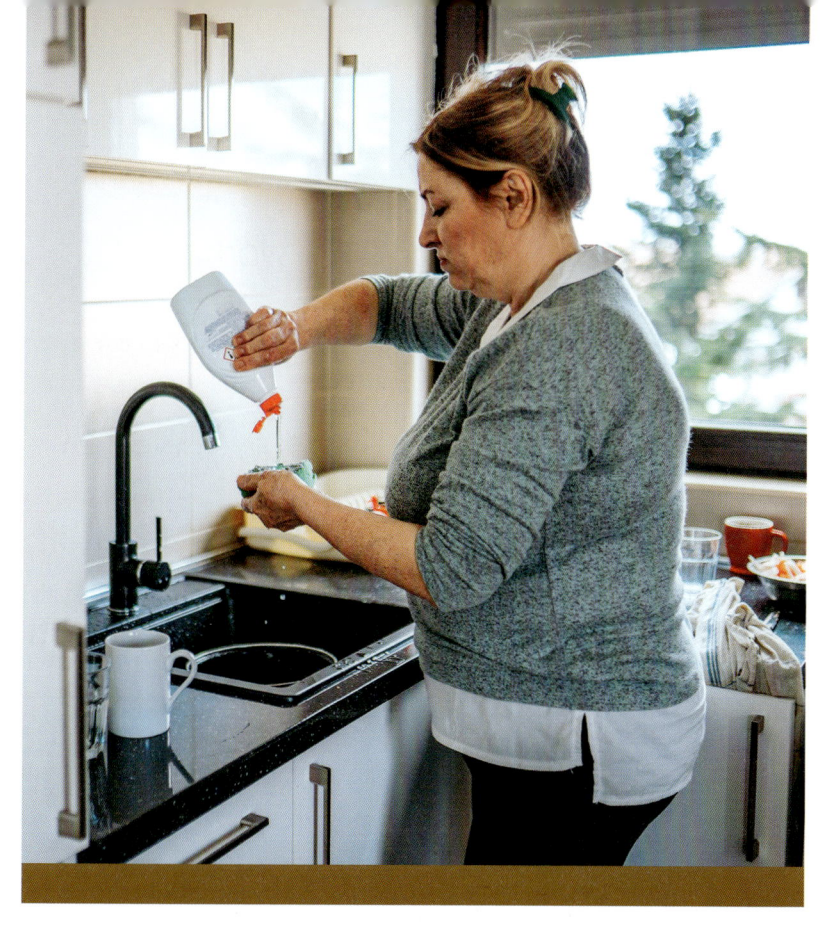

Sometimes, home health aides need to do some light housekeeping, which might include washing the dishes.

in and out of bed. Student aides also learn how to help patients exercise. Another ten hours of the course is dedicated to housekeeping. Student aides learn to clean a patient's home. They learn home safety, laundry, and more. However, working health aides are not maids. Marisol Rivera is an aide with more than twenty years of experience. She told the *Guardian*, "One of the biggest challenges is explaining that you are not a maid. That your job is not to clean up after everyone."[2]

Learning about patient nutrition is an important part of training. Aides in California need sixteen hours of learning. They learn about food and cooking. They are trained to keep cookware and dishes clean and sanitary. They also learn how to store food properly.

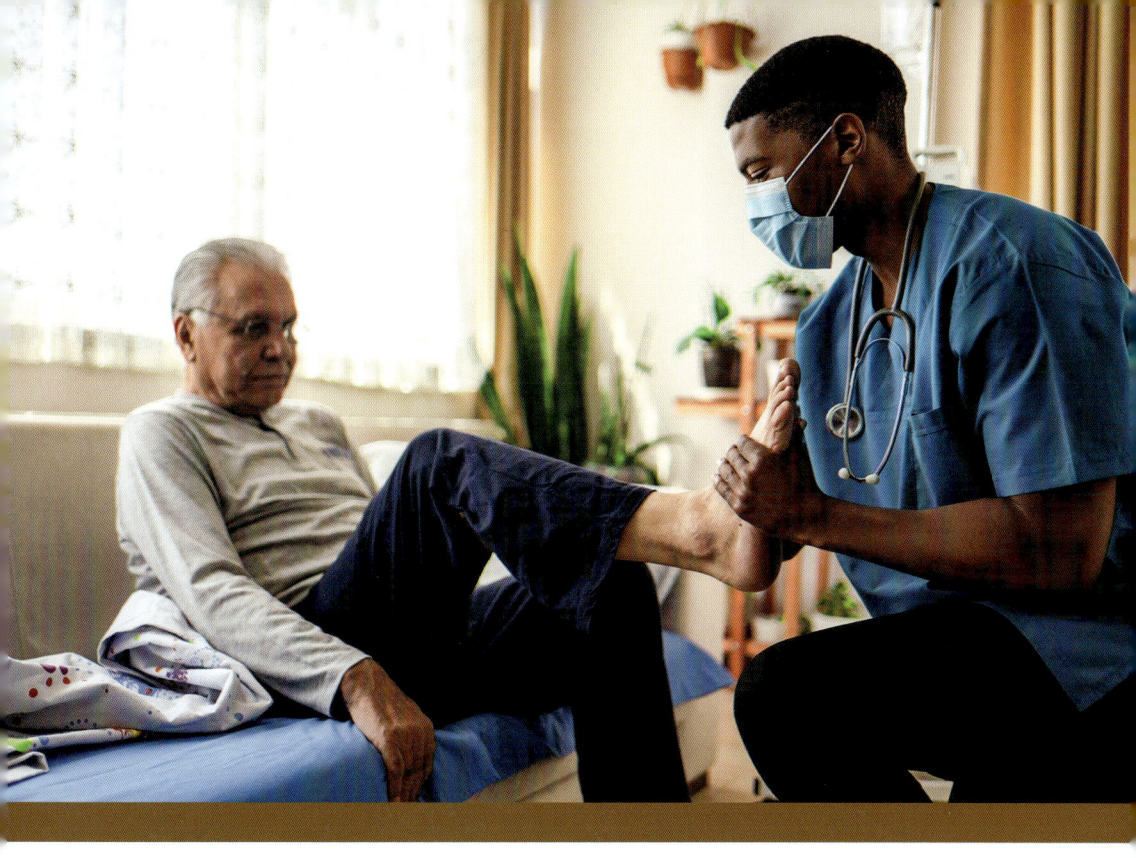

Physical therapists can teach home health aides how to help patients with basic stretching.

Registered nurses often do most of the personal care training. Other specialists might lead different parts of the coursework. Physical therapists can teach aides about mobility and exercise. Nutritionists and social workers can teach students in their subject areas. Social workers help aides relate to their patients and their needs.

ADDITIONAL TRAINING AND SKILLS

Training and certification are the first steps in a career as a home health aide. Aides need to continue learning if they want better and higher-paying jobs. Many states require additional training once a year. This could mean taking a course to brush up on one's skills. The training might address new requirements. These are established by organizations like the NAHC or by federal or state laws.

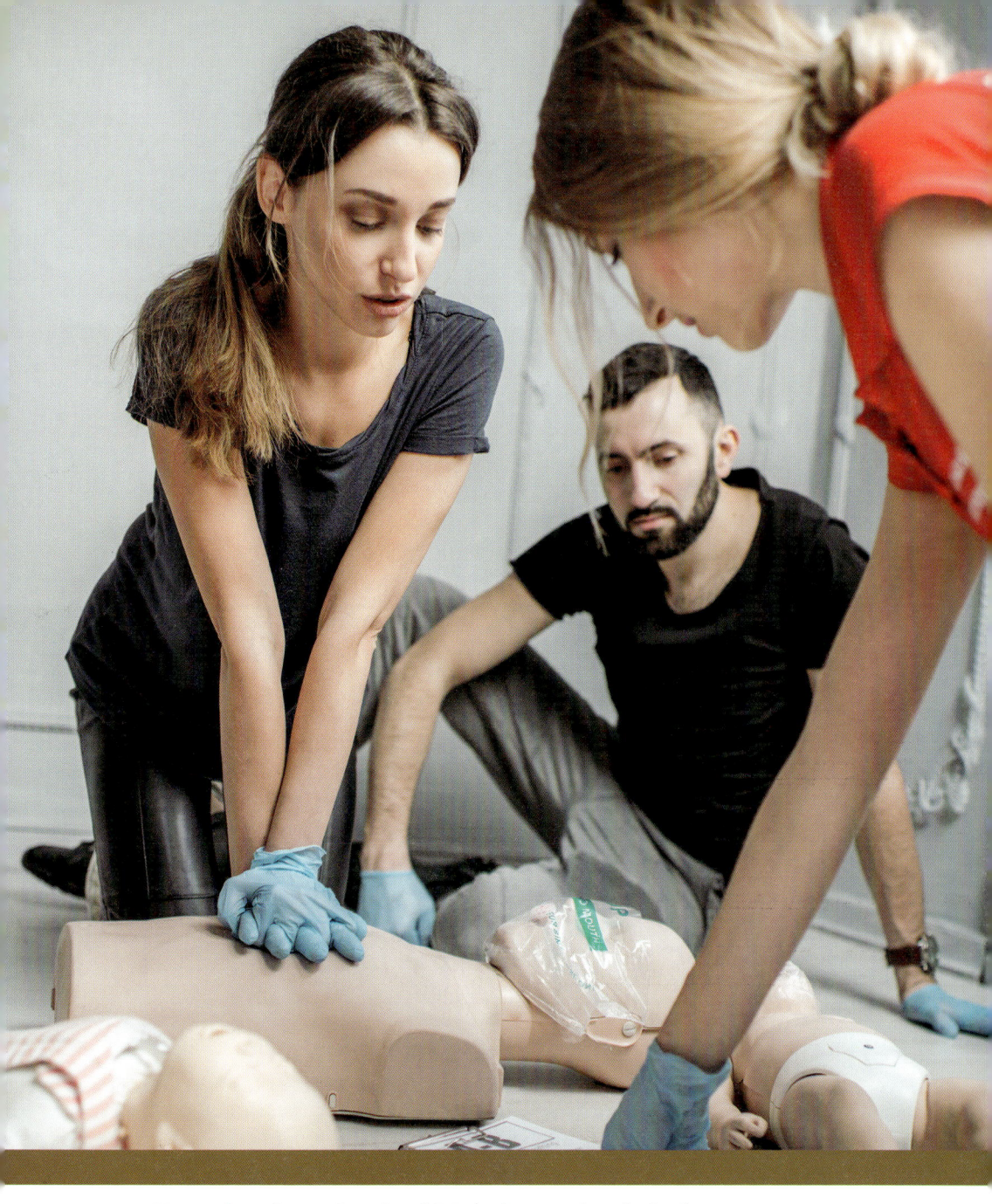

Knowing how to do CPR is important during emergency situations.

Every state has its own rules on annual training and class requirements. The state of Florida's Agency for Health Care Administration (AHCA) makes all home health aides get certifications in **CPR**. They must also take an HIV/AIDS training course once a year.

As they move forward in their careers, aides often get more training and certifications. They can then use special equipment like ventilators to help with breathing. Some patients might need emergency tools, such as an automated external defibrillator (AED). This is a portable

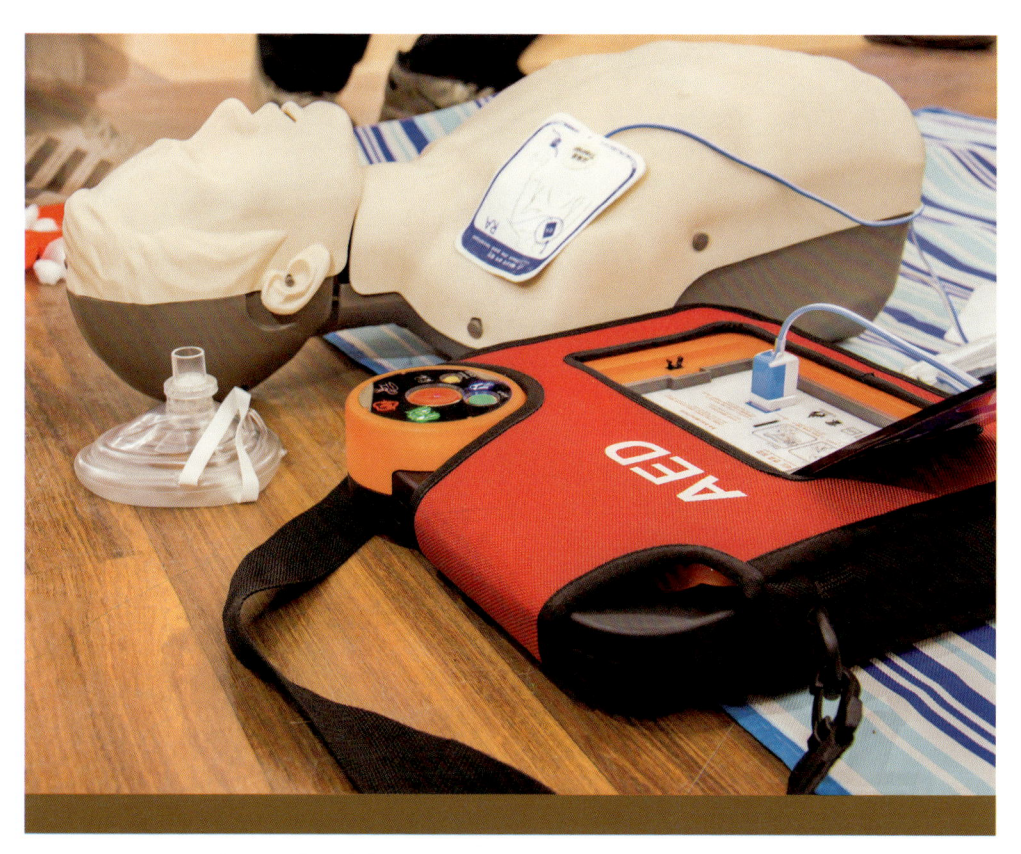

Home health aides can get training to use a defibrillator.

device. It helps shock a patient's heart back to a normal rhythm if their heart stops. Health aides can also get training to help patients with special needs. For example, aides can specialize in caring for elderly

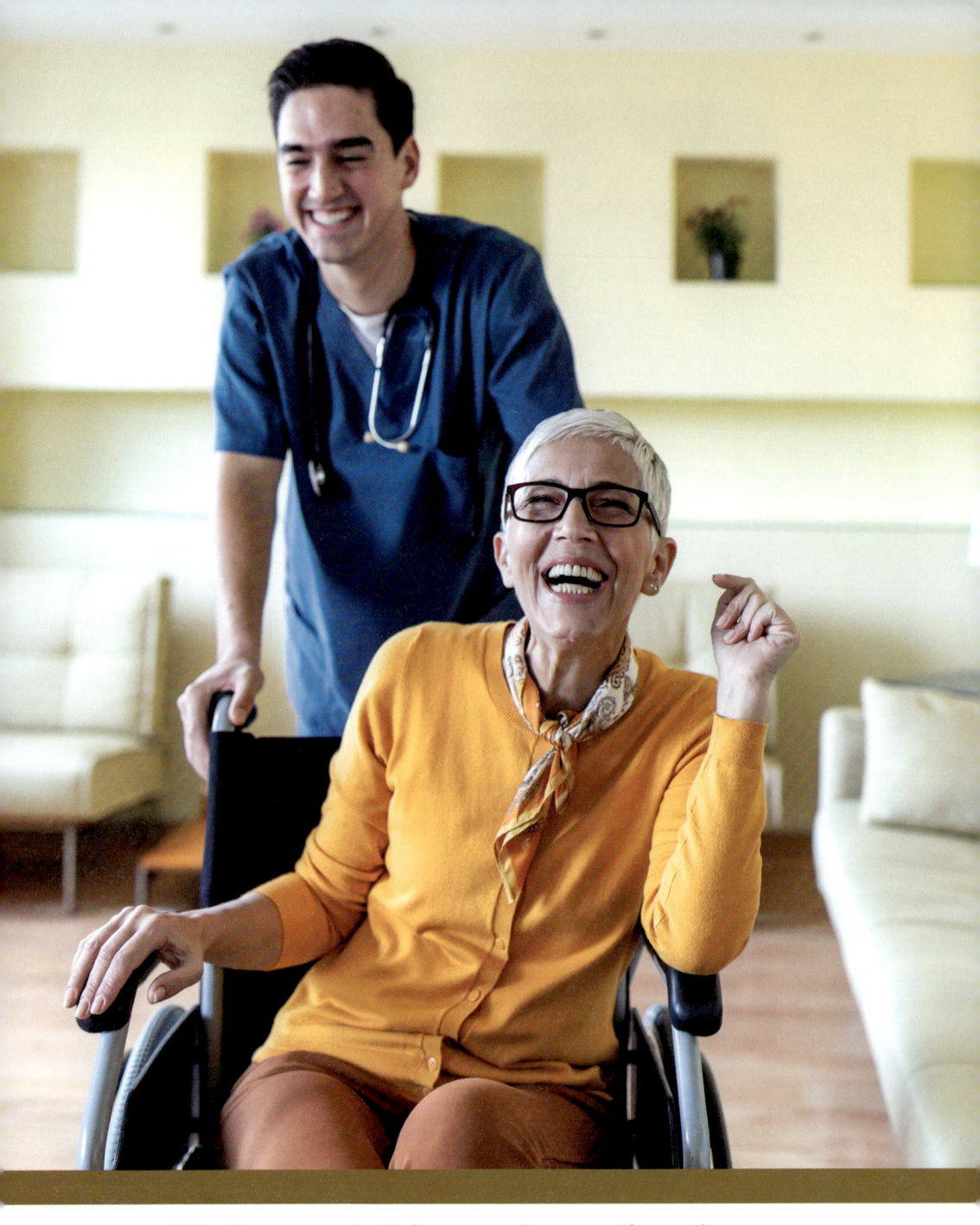

Offering more trainings and promotions does not help only the health aide. Patients also benefit from a health aide who is well prepared and happy.

patients. They can specialize in clients with heart conditions or behavioral issues.

Stephen McCall of the Public Health Institute says that when training offers a clear career path, it can attract more aides. Many workers work for years with only small pay increases. Such workers rarely get a promotion. McCall told National Public Radio (NPR), "It means that their skills that they're developing over time, providing services to older adults and people with disabilities, often go unrecognized and unrewarded."[3]

CHAPTER THREE

WHAT IS LIFE LIKE AS A HOME HEALTH AIDE?

A health aide with several patients often starts the day at their agency. They meet with their patients' nurses or doctors. They might discuss their patients' change in medication. Meetings can also be about whether their patient needs extra care and preparation.

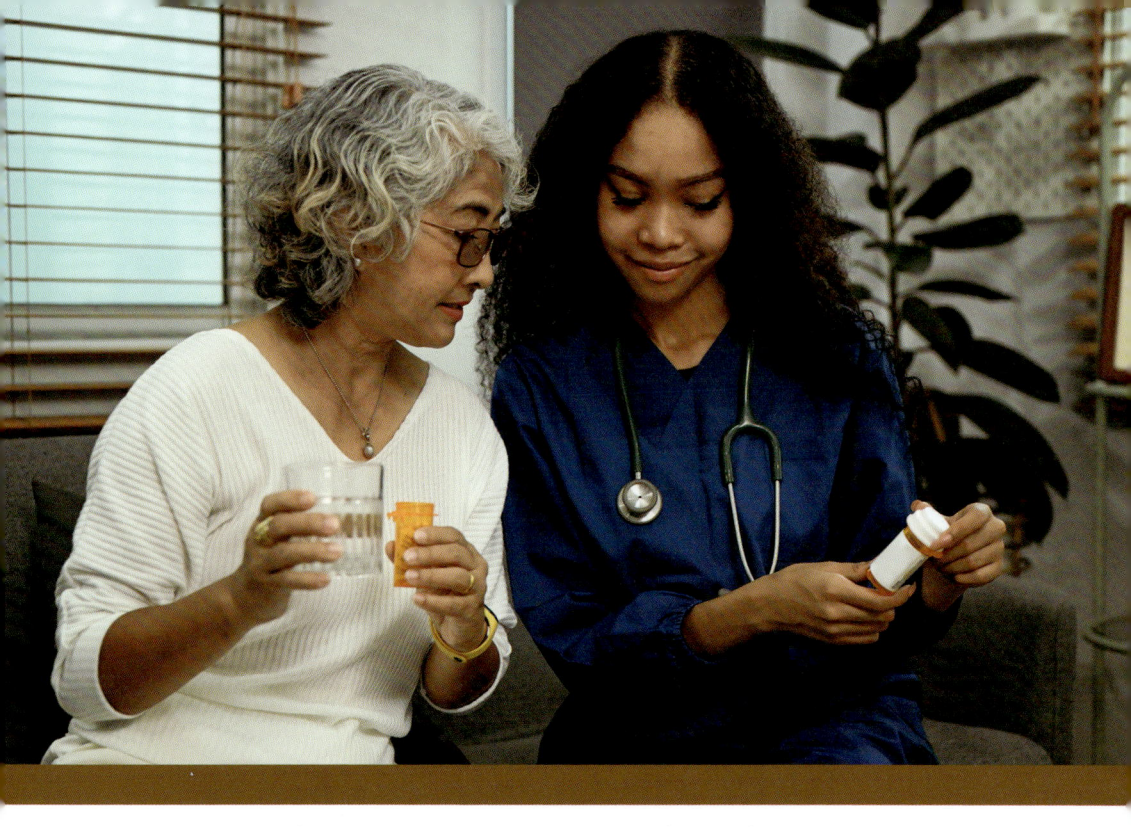

Health aides must make sure their patients are taking the right kind of medication at the right time.

The aide's duties vary depending on the time of day. The first shift of the day can involve helping a patient get out of bed. Health aides may need to help the patient bathe. They can help patients brush their teeth. If the patient is able, the aide may

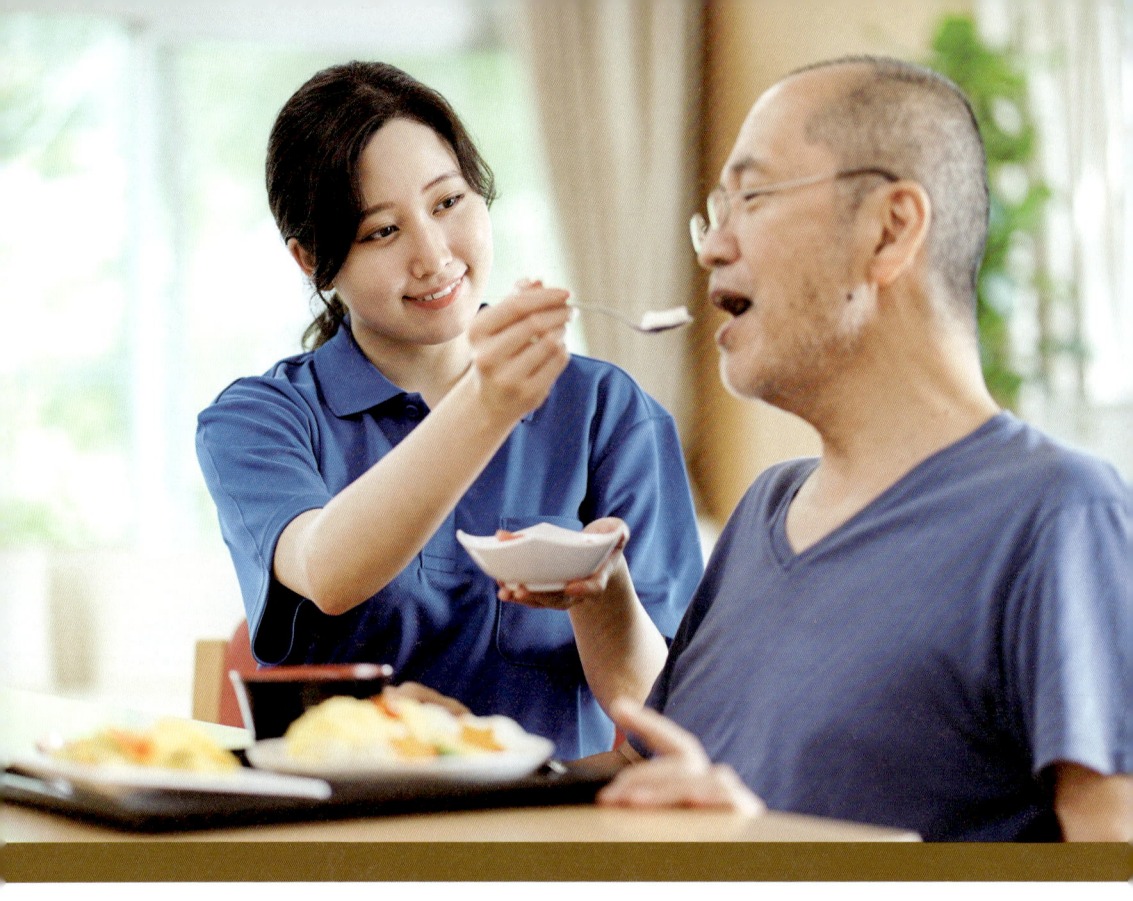

Some health aides need to help their patients eat their daily meals.

help them take a walk. Aides may help them stretch or exercise. They can help a patient's muscle or joint pain with massage.

Then an aide might cook breakfast for their patient. They might also prepare meals for the rest of the day or week. If needed, they will take a patient grocery shopping or go shopping for them. An aide who visits different patients throughout the day will cover different ADLs and IADLs. Whatever their tasks, most health aides need to develop certain skills.

SKILLS OF A HOME HEALTH AIDE

The skills and training aides get are just the beginning. Many health aides are their patient's main source of human contact. Live-in aides can become even closer to their patients than family.

Communication is essential. Aides must be able to talk to clients who are difficult or mentally unwell. Health aides must also give nurses and doctors accurate information. Patients' families and other caregivers need similar updates.

Aides must be observant. They need to be detail oriented. They must ask the right questions to make sure their patient feels well. This includes understanding their patient's body language. It also includes noticing changes in the patient's condition. The aide must react well to emergencies or other problems.

Health aides handle messes and situations that others might find unpleasant.

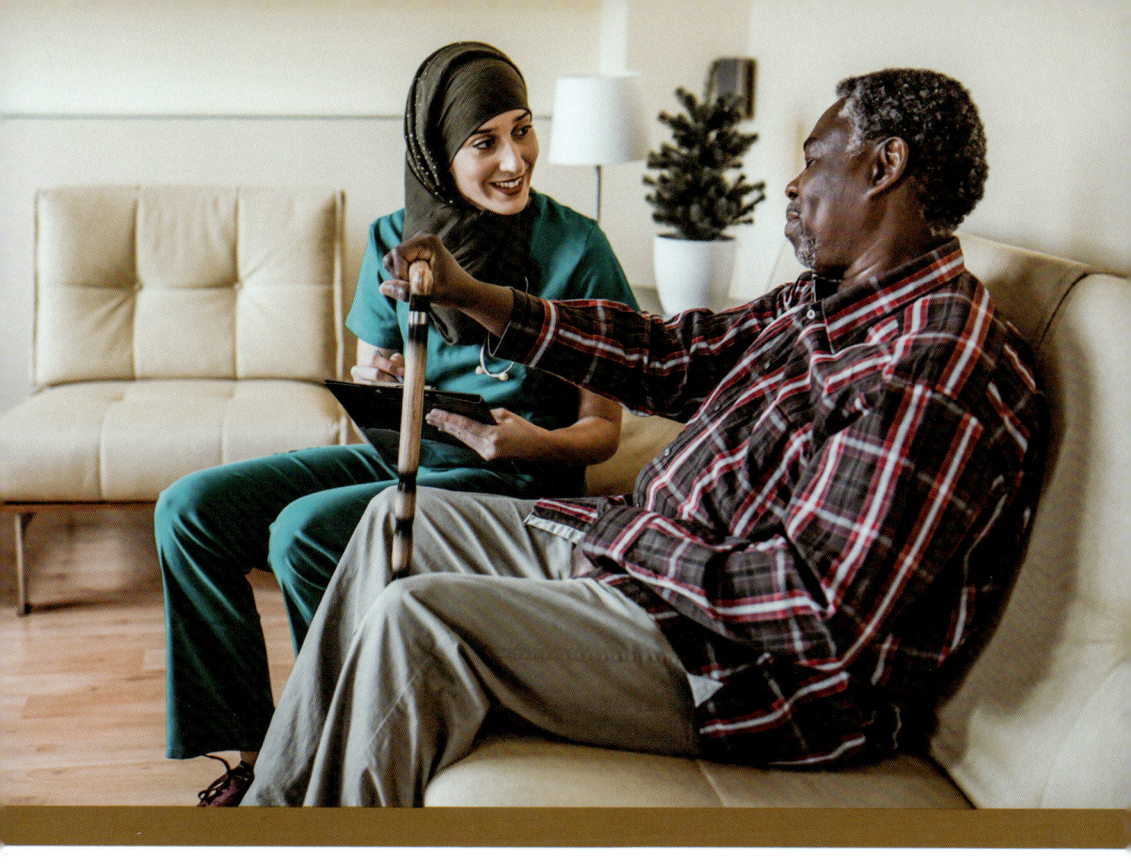

Health aides are great communicators. They must stay connected with patients, as well as the patient's family members and other health care providers.

For example, some patients cannot control when they go to the bathroom. They must wear adult diapers or pads. These must be changed out on time. Patients also need help cleaning themselves. A home health aide named May worked her job for eleven years. She had about 100 elderly clients in total. Some were very sick, and many were unable to care for themselves at all. "They couldn't move at all," May said. "I had to change them, feed them, bathe them, everything."[4]

    Health aides sometimes work with patients who have unstable emotions and mental health issues. For example, patients with Alzheimer's disease or dementia can act out. They may not be able to control their emotions, words, or actions. Aides must be patient. They need to be able to

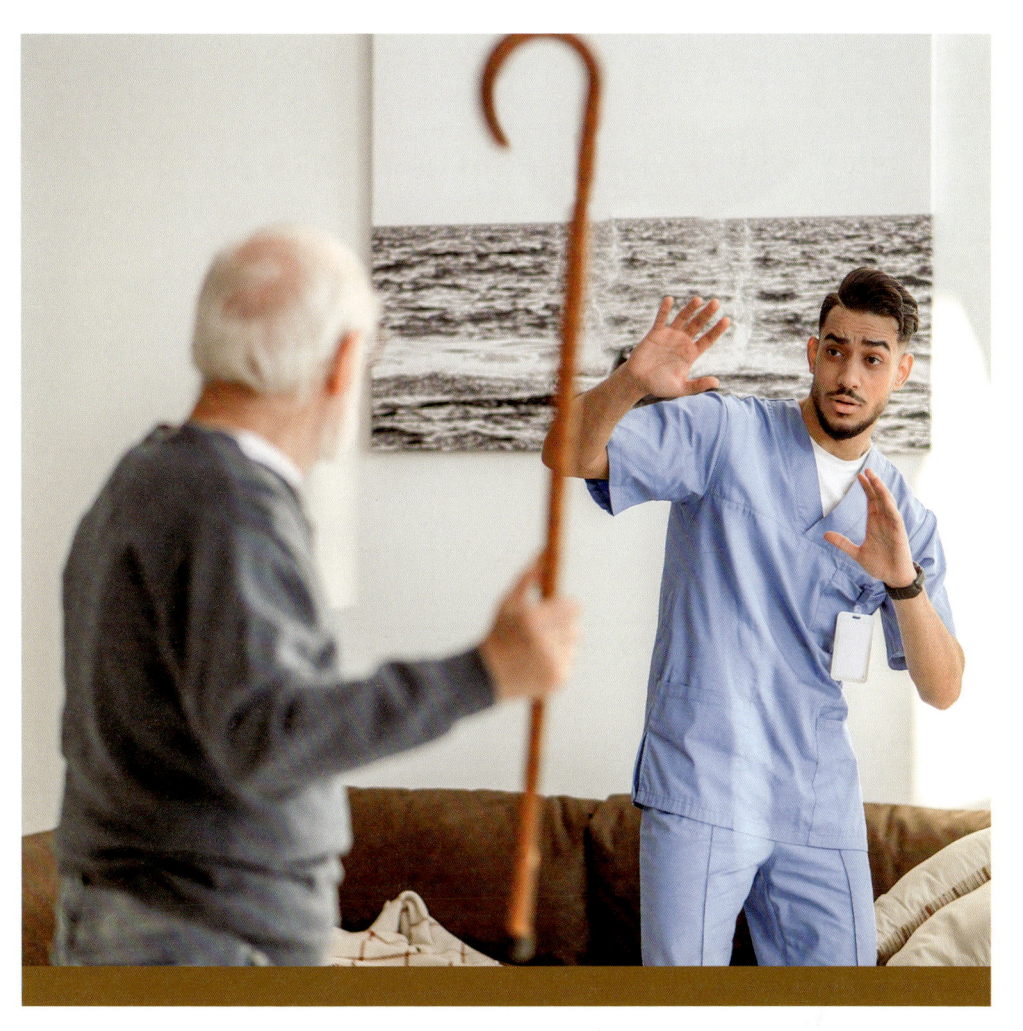

Aides must know how to be patient and calm when working with people who cannot control their emotions or actions.

manage the situation. Patients with wild

mood swings can be stressful to deal

with. Aides must learn not to take abusive

language or actions personally. At the same time, they must judge whether it is safe to be around particular patients. For live-in aides, dealing with such issues is an around-the-clock job.

Aides also must have good physical strength. For example, patients with Parkinson's disease or paralysis must be moved around. Aides receive training on how best to move a patient from a bed to a wheelchair. They do this to keep the patient safe. They also must look after their own safety. Being careless can easily lead to injuries.

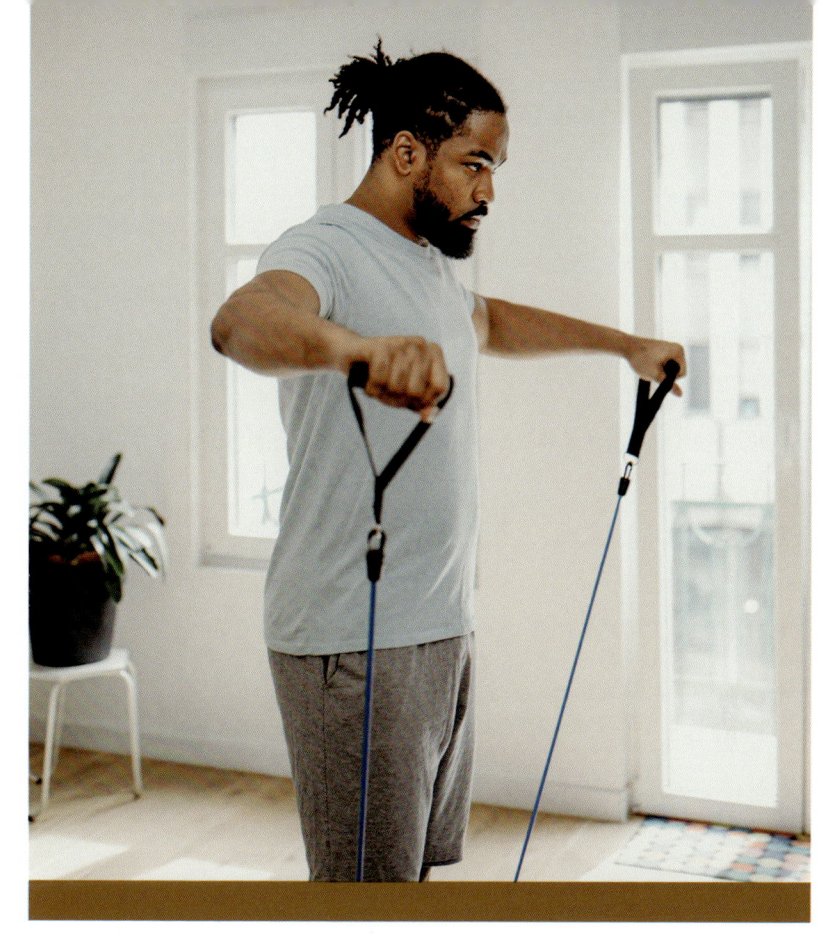

It is important for aides to take care of their own health so they don't get sick or injured on the job.

THE HUMAN TOUCH

Health aides provide companionship. Many patients do not have family or friends to help or visit them. Health aides are more than just workers to these patients.

They can also be friends. Aides might be the only people they regularly see. This human contact is very important for patients. It helps their physical and mental health. Loneliness and depression are common for many patients. These mental health conditions can raise blood pressure. They can also make Alzheimer's, heart issues, and other problems worse.

Patients are not the only ones who feel this human connection. A big part of the job is the satisfaction health aides get from helping others. Home health aide Debra Blank works in Maryland.

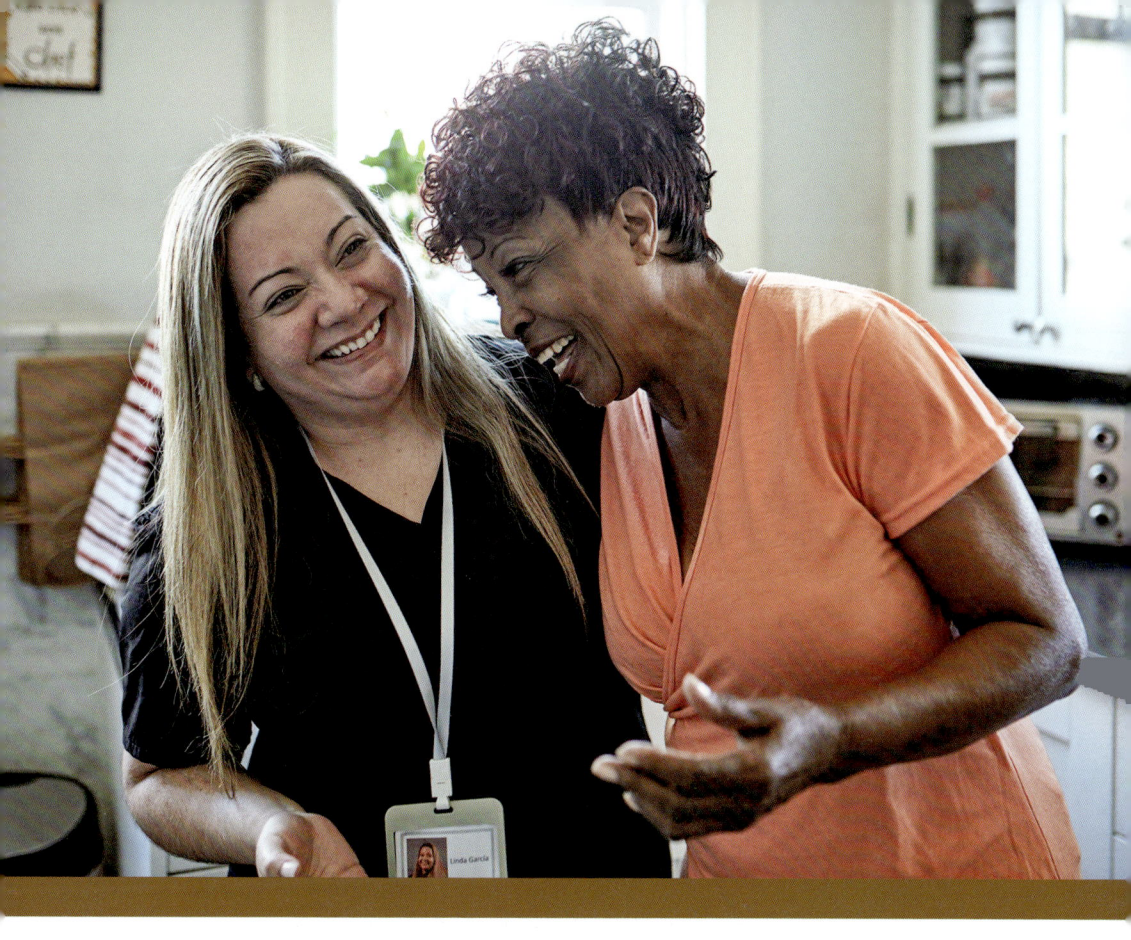

For many patients, home health aides are more than just caretakers.

She told Care.com about how her job was rewarding. Helping others made her happy. "Even if I only change one person's life, it makes me feel so good to know I've done something to help someone, because there are so many people out there who need help," she said. "This work just makes you feel so good about yourself, and you're showing other people that you care about them and you're compassionate for them."[5]

GEARING UP, STAYING EQUIPPED

The federal government, states, and home health agencies have different rules on what equipment health aides are allowed to use. This often depends on training and certifications. Health aides usually cannot handle specialized medical equipment. However, they can use blood pressure and pulse monitors. They can also use

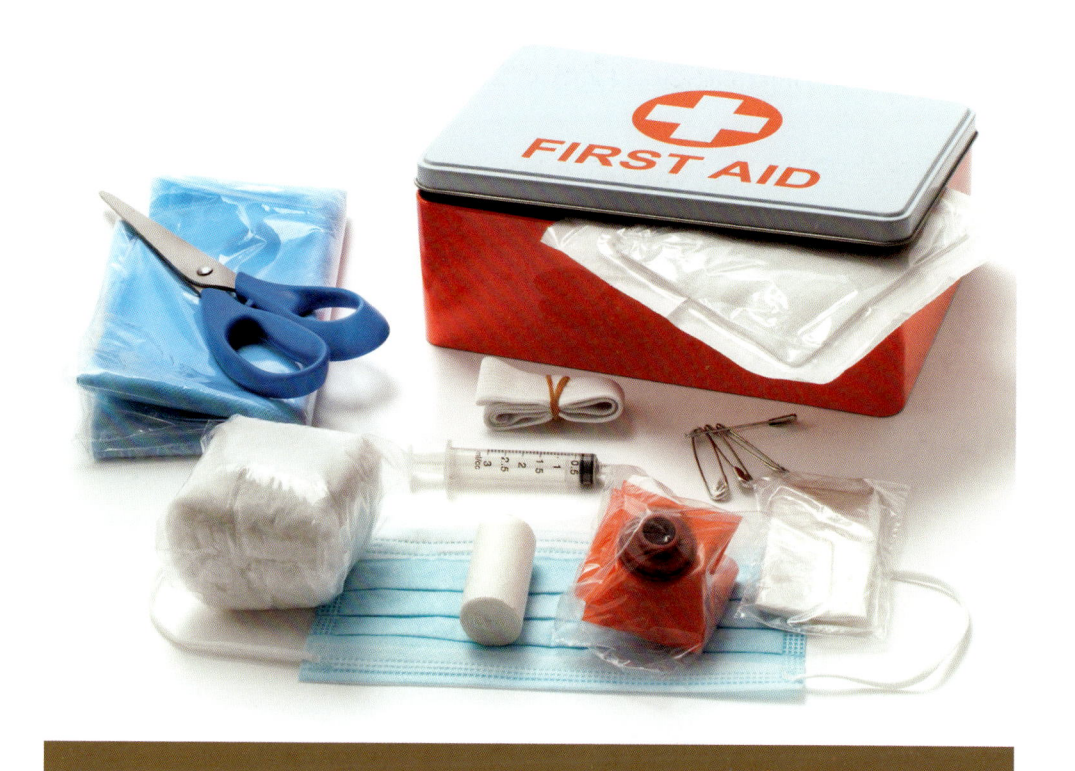

Health aides must know how to use first aid equipment.

thermometers. Aides can handle wound care by providing bandages. They can also adjust and clean **catheters** and similar equipment.

Cold and warm compresses and hot water bottles are some items aides may use. First-aid creams and ointments are also common tools. Aides should also know how to handle wheelchairs, crutches, and walkers.

Aides can use a work bag to keep commonly used items handy. Ben Nelson wrote an article for healthcare staffing company Anodyne. Nelson had several tips for health aides regarding work bags. He wrote, "An over-the-shoulder or crossbody strap allows you to carry your bag and keep both hands free . . . You need to quickly locate frequently used items such as pens, hand sanitizer, and your phone. Thus, look for a bag with at least a few zipper pockets and/or compartments. After all, you don't want to spend your day digging through your bag."[6]

CAREGIVING IN THE AGE OF COVID

The COVID-19 pandemic affected the jobs of health aides. Many patients had conditions that made them more vulnerable to the virus. Aides needed to wear face masks and gloves. They also had to wash their hands many times a day. Aides had to be careful at all times. Passing the virus to their already weakened patients could be dangerous.

CHAPTER FOUR

WHAT IS THE FUTURE FOR HOME HEALTH AIDES?

The number of health aides exploded in the early 2000s. In 2019, the *New York Times* reported that there had been a 150 percent growth in home care workers in the previous ten years. By 2019 there were about 2.3 million. This number covered all

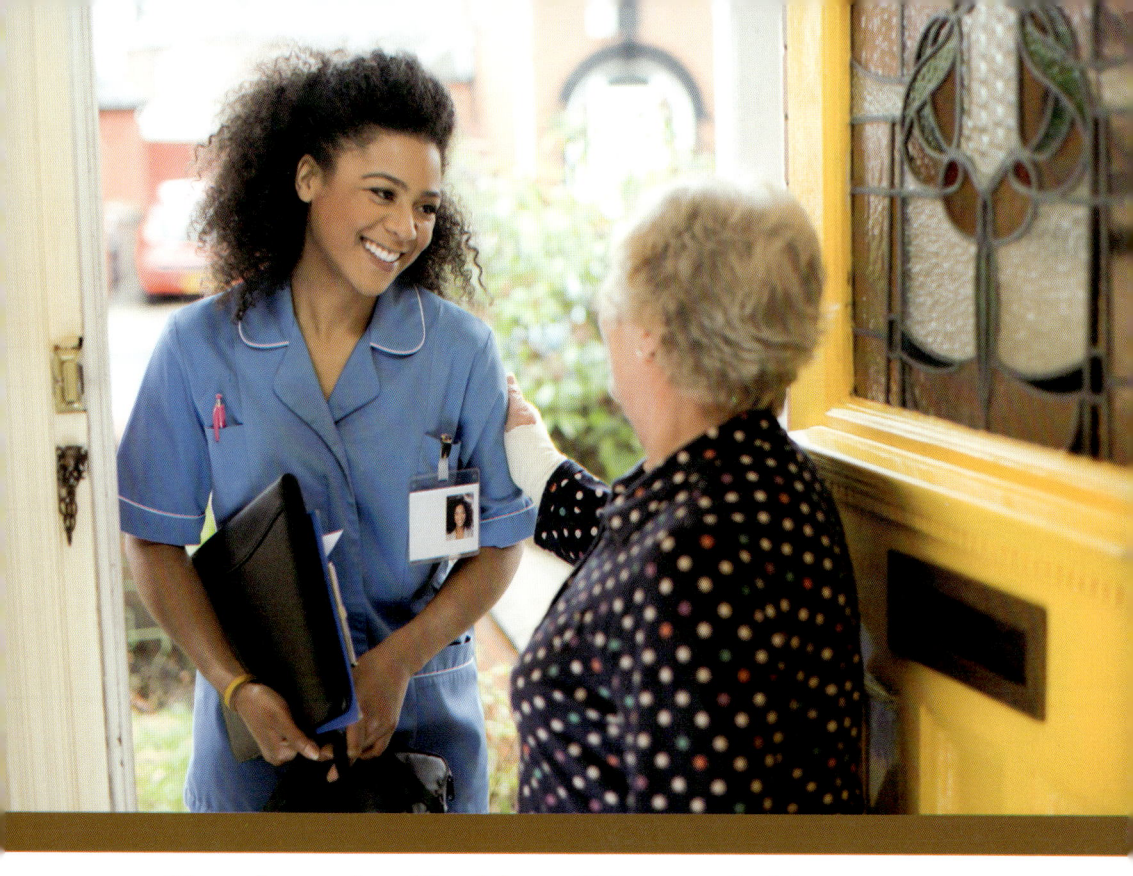

More home health aides will be needed in the future.

home caregivers. Other experts noted that only a small portion of this total were health aides. Career site Zippia estimated that 314,565 were home health aides.

NPR noted that the number of Americans sixty and older will increase by 30 percent by 2050. The Bureau of Labor Statistics (BLS) predicts that home health aides will be needed more than ever. Job openings are expected to rise by 37 percent by 2028. In 2022, there were not enough aides working to cover the many thousands of people that needed them.

Many poor, older Americans qualify for Medicare. This money could pay for health aides. But thousands are on waiting lists. Agencies and organizations cannot fill the jobs. University of Ohio economics professor John Bowblis pointed out to NPR how this hurts the poor. He said, "If you're

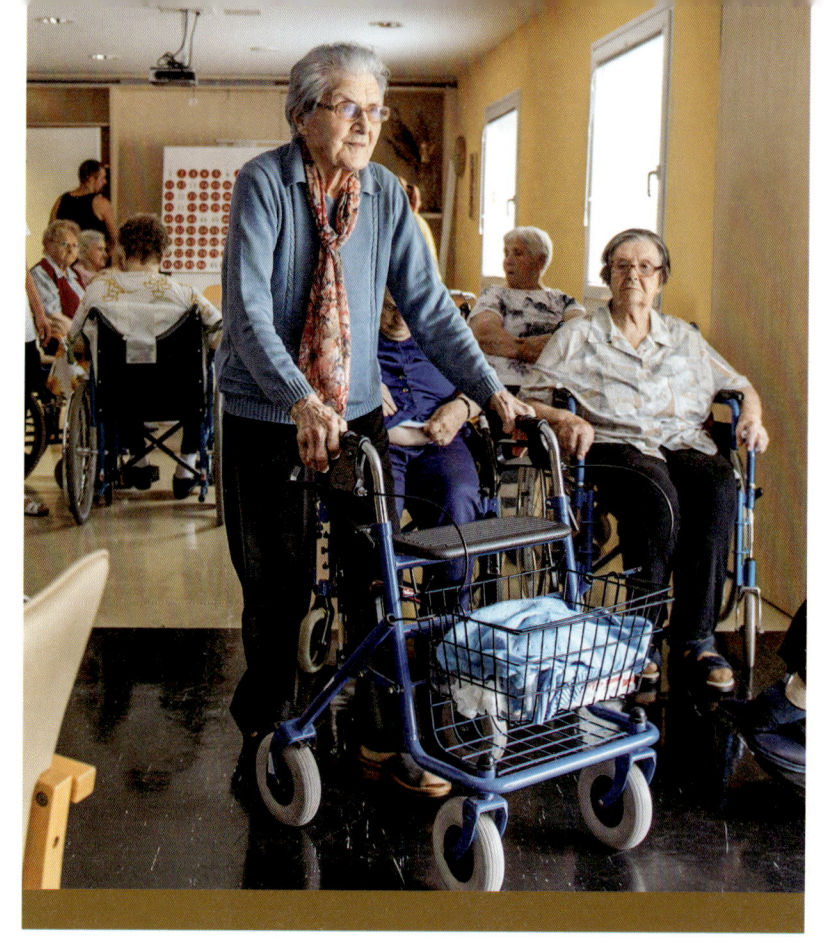

Seniors who do not have home health aides may have to stay in nursing homes or hospitals.

somebody on Medicaid, you don't have those financial resources. . . . And the only solution is to basically force someone to go into congregate living, like an assisted living or nursing home, or you're going to be on a waiting list."[7] Government programs pay less for health aides. In Indiana, the state's Medicaid program only covers health aide pay up to $13 an hour.

HEALTH AIDES DURING THE PANDEMIC

The COVID-19 pandemic started in 2020. It had many negative effects on health care in the United States. Health aides faced many difficulties. Doing their jobs put their own health at risk. Patients also risked getting COVID-19 from their caregivers.

Health aides visiting several clients had to be very careful. Between every visit, they had to change their uniforms and personal

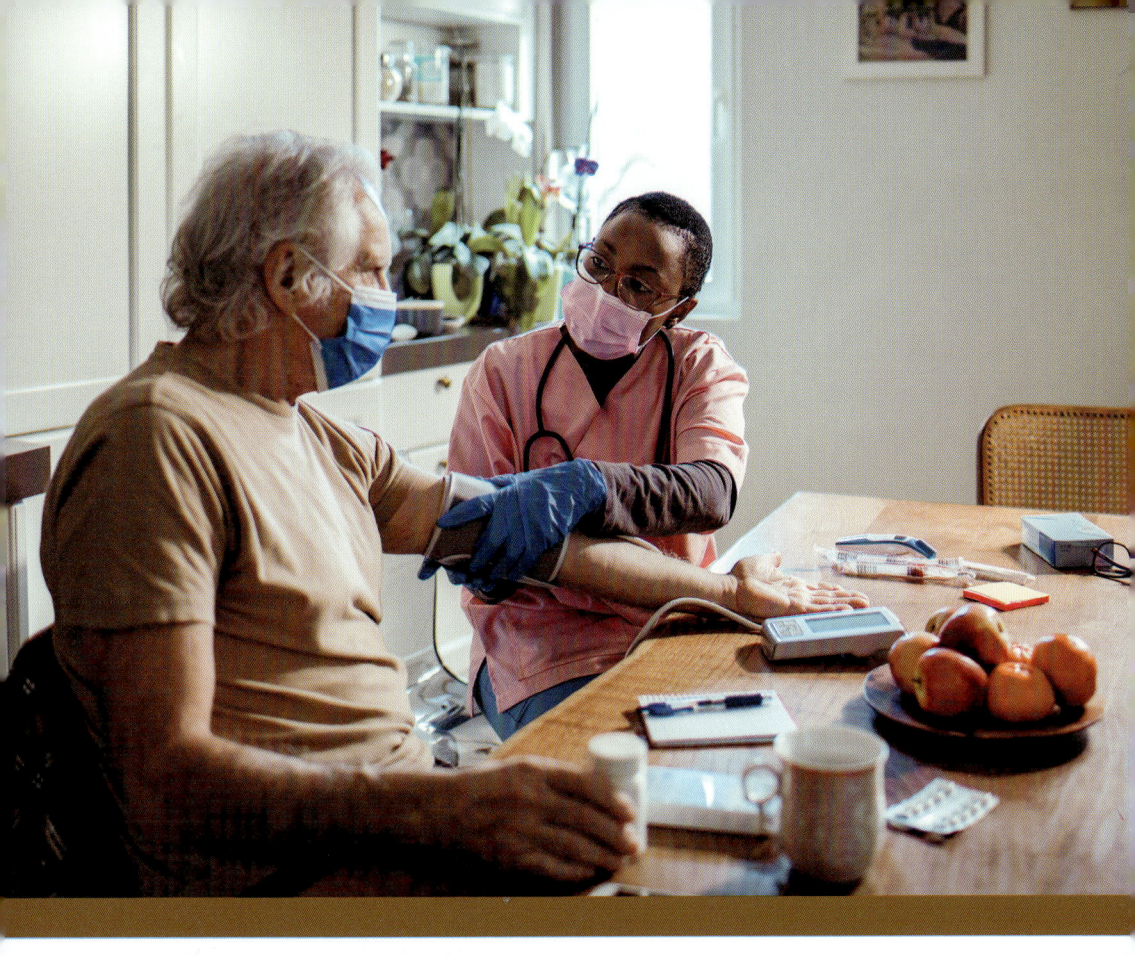

During the pandemic, home health aides had to be very careful about their health and the health of their patients. Wearing masks and gloves helped.

protective equipment (PPE). PPE includes masks, gloves, and protective body suits. When the pandemic started, there was a shortage of PPE. Aides risked their lives as COVID-19 spread. The virus affected elderly patients the hardest. The pandemic showed the challenge of being a home health aide. The fear of the virus made many health aides quit.

BURNOUT AND RESPECT

The future of the health aide field is complicated. Many people like the job

A TRAGEDY ON THE FRONT LINES

Sue Williams-Ward was a home health aide in Indianapolis, Indiana. When one of her patients showed symptoms of COVID-19, Williams-Ward asked for PPE. However, her agency never gave it. Ward ended up getting COVID-19 from her patient. She spent weeks in the hospital. Some weeks were spent on a ventilator. Ward died of COVID-19 at age 68.

because they like helping others. But many aides are tired of the low pay. It doesn't help that the work hours are long and difficult. Many health aides get little respect for doing such a tough and important job. This is why **burnout** is common among aides. The conditions of the pandemic only made burnout worse.

Thalia, a health aide, quit her job because of COVID-19. But she had other reasons to leave, too. At one point she hurt her foot. Her job didn't provide health insurance. She couldn't pay for physical therapy. This forced her out of work for months.

The stress of working for one particular client also got to Thalia. "Sometimes," she explained, "the kitchen would be a disaster, and in order for me to get her meals prepared, I would have to clean up the mess that was left by the family members."[8] She also had patients' families asking her to do their laundry and housekeeping. Though this work was not part of her job, she felt pressured. She worried the families would ask her agency to replace her.

In 2021, the BLS said that home health aides had a **median income** of $29,430. University of Pennsylvania professor Rachel

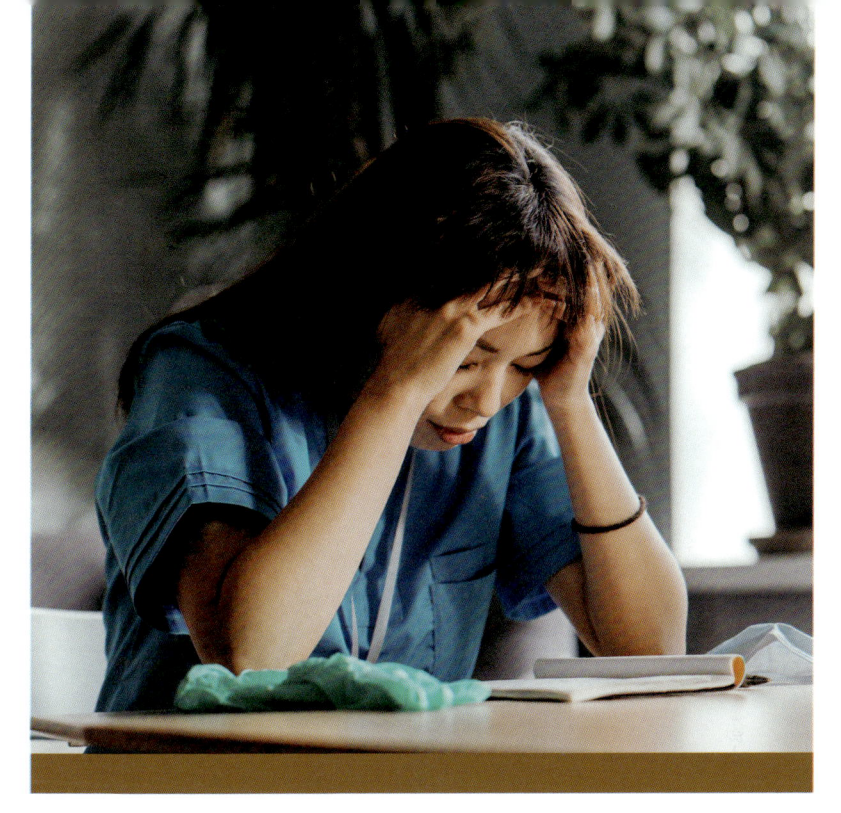

The pandemic shed light on how home health aides received low pay compared to how much work they did.

Werner studies the health care industry. She pointed out how the gender and ethnicity of health aides affected their salaries and status. Almost all health aides were women. More than half were non-white. "Statistics like this really help describe a workforce that doesn't have a lot of political capital," says Werner. "And so they're a pretty vulnerable workforce."[9]

IMPROVING THE INDUSTRY

It is likely that many future patients will suffer from this worker shortage. Improving the jobs of health aides could attract more workers. Health aides in all states could also get more training. The more skilled a worker is, the more they tend to earn.

For example, many states do not let health aides change bandages or give out medication directly. These jobs are done by nurses. And the jobs are often done in

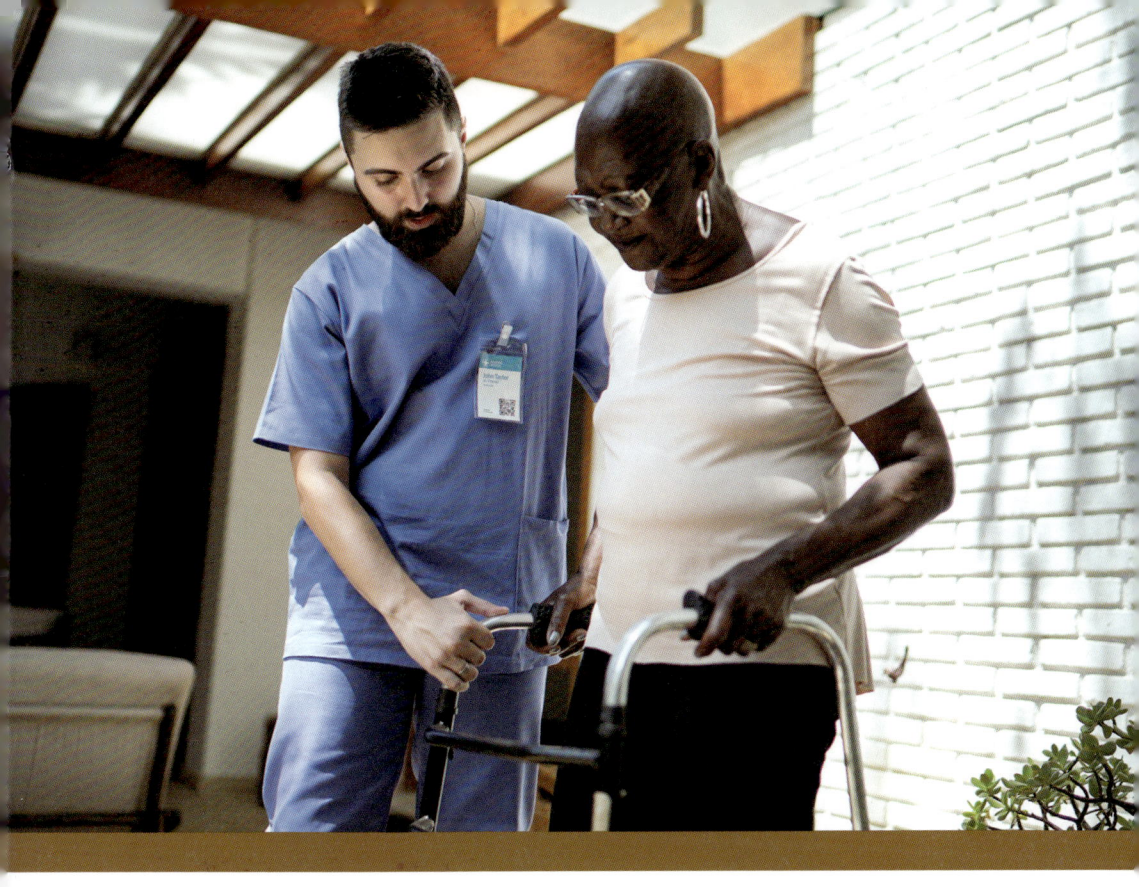

The health care industry needs more skilled health aides.

clinics or hospitals. A lot of money could be saved by letting health aides take over some of these tasks. More government money is also needed. This money could fund better training for aides. It could also help with pay raises.

THE OUTLOOK FOR HEALTH AIDES

Home health aides will be an important part of health care for many years to come. Many health aides on the job today are middle-aged or older. More positions will open as workers retire or quit.

As the need for these workers grows, it is important to improve their pay and work conditions. Without these steps, many patients will go without the care they need. Government funding and new laws can help. Better pay and more respect for health aides can go a long way. These improvements will make it a career that will

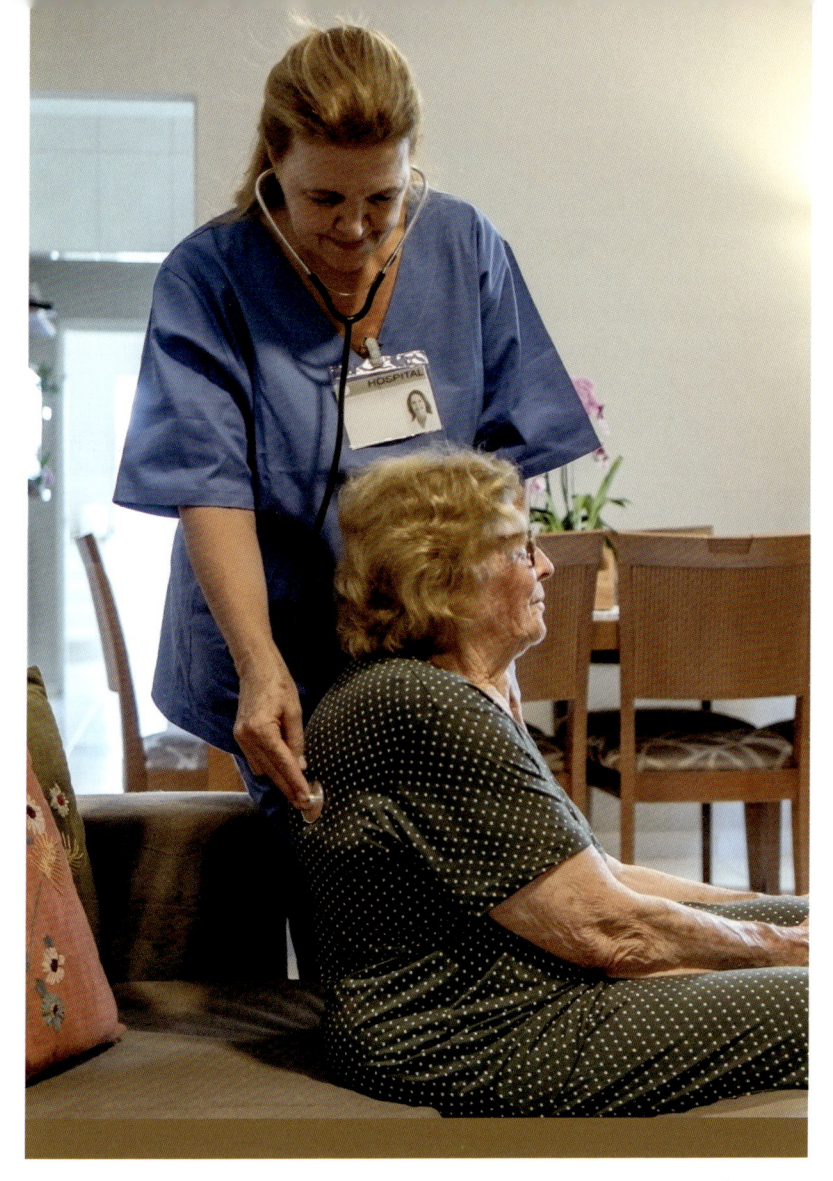

Advocates argue that the government and private agencies need to improve home health aide working conditions.

attract the caring and dedicated people

patients need.

GLOSSARY

burnout
the feeling of being exhausted from doing a job

catheter
a medical tube that is put into the human body to allow for injections or to remove fluids, like urine from the bladder

CPR
stands for cardiopulmonary resuscitation, a technique that can save a person's life if their heart stops

entry-level
describing a job that someone takes at the beginning of a career, when they have little or no work experience

hygiene
the practice of keeping one's body clean and appearance presentable

median income
the middle point of income ranges for a particular job or profession

mobility aids
any tools or equipment that help disabled people get around

vulnerable
describing a person or group that is less able to protect themselves from harm or danger

SOURCE NOTES

CHAPTER ONE: WHAT DOES A HEALTH AIDE DO?

1. Quoted in Milli Legrain, "Why Do One in Five Home Health Aides Live in Poverty?" *Guardian*, September 18, 2019. www.theguardian.com.

CHAPTER TWO: WHAT TRAINING DO HOME HEALTH AIDES NEED?

2. Quoted in Legrain, "Why Do One in Five Home Health Aides Live in Poverty?"

3. Quoted in Natalie Krebs, "A Shortage of Health Aides Is Forcing Out Those Who Wish to Get Care at Home," *NPR*, May 5, 2022. www.npr.org.

CHAPTER THREE: WHAT IS LIFE LIKE AS A HOME HEALTH AIDE?

4. Quoted in Kavitha Cardoza, "'We're Aides, Not Maids.' How One High-Demand Job Shows Education System's Failings," *Hechinger Report*, October 7, 2021. https://hechingerreport.org.

5. Quoted in Emily Starbuck Gerson, "How to Become a Certified Home Health Aide," *Care.com*, April 13, 2022. www.care.com.

6. Quoted in Ben Nelson, "What's in Your Bag? How to Prepare for a Day as a Home Health Aide," September 13, 2021. www.anodyne-services.com.

CHAPTER FOUR: WHAT IS THE FUTURE FOR HOME HEALTH AIDES?

7. Quoted in Krebs, "A Shortage of Health Aides Is Forcing Out Those Who Wish to Get Care at Home."

8. Quoted in Cardoza, "'We're Aides, Not Maids.' How One High-Demand Job Shows Education System's Failings."

9. Quoted in Krebs, "A Shortage of Health Aides Is Forcing Out Those Who Wish to Get Care at Home."

FOR FURTHER RESEARCH

BOOKS

Emma Huddleston, *Work in the Health Care Industry*. San Diego, CA: BrightPoint Press, 2020.

Wendy Hinote Lanier, *Become a Physical Therapy Assistant*. San Diego, CA: BrightPoint Press, 2023.

Martha London, *The Spread of COVID-19*. Minneapolis, MN: Abdo Publishing, 2021.

INTERNET SOURCES

Andy Newman, "On the Job, 24 Hours a Day, 27 Days a Month," *New York Times*, September 2, 2019. www.nytimes.com.

"Occupational Outlook Handbook: Home Health and Personal Care Aides," *US Bureau of Labor Statistics (BLS)*, September 8, 2022. www.bls.gov.

"What Is a Health Aide?" *Zippia*, n.d. www.zippia.com.

WEBSITES

Home Care Association of America
www.hcaoa.org

The Home Care Association of America is a trade organization made up of home care agencies and their suppliers and vendors.

National Association for Home Care & Hospice (NAHC)
www.nahc.org

The National Association for Home Care & Hospice (NAHC) is the main professional association dedicated to caregivers and their patients. Its membership is made up of the many private companies, nonprofit and governmental institutions, workers, and educators in the industry.

Public Health Institute
www.phi.org

The Public Health Institute is a national nonprofit organization that works to improve the system of home health care for both workers and patients. It helps lawmakers work on these issues and is involved in improving teaching and training for direct care workers.

INDEX

ADLs, 17–18, 21, 47
agencies, 16, 28, 30–31, 40, 44, 56, 62, 66, 68
Agency for Health Care Administration (AHCA), 40
Alzheimer's disease, 8, 50, 54

Blank, Debra, 54
Bowblis, John, 62
Bureau of Labor Statistics (BLS), 62, 68

certifications, 28, 31, 33, 38, 40, 56
COVID-19 pandemic, 59, 64–67

dementia, 50
Dettmer, Bob, 6–8
doctors, 12, 14, 24–25, 44, 48

Graduate Educational Development (GED), 26–28

housekeeping, 19, 28, 35, 68

IADLs, 19–21, 47

live-in aides, 8, 16, 47, 52

May, 50
McCall, Stephen, 43
Medicaid, 16, 31, 32, 63–64
medical equipment, 24, 40, 56–58
Medicare, 16, 31, 32, 62
medications, 20, 22–23, 25, 44, 70
mental health, 50, 54

National Association for Home Care & Hospice (NAHC), 31, 33, 38
National Public Radio (NPR), 43, 61, 63
Nelson, Ben, 58
New York Times, 8, 60
nonprofit organizations, 16, 33
nurses, 8, 12, 14, 24–25, 37, 44, 48, 71

O'Bryant, Deborah, 18

Parkinson's disease, 7, 52
personal protective equipment (PPE), 65, 66

Rivera, Marisol, 36

Salmon, Marjorie, 6–8

Thalia, 67–68
training, 28–30, 32, 34, 36–43, 47, 52, 56, 70, 72

vocational schools, 28, 33

Werner, Rachel, 69–70
Williams-Ward, Sue, 66
work conditions, 72

IMAGE CREDITS

Cover: © kali9/iStockphoto
5: © Magdalena Juillard/Shutterstock Images
7: © FG Trade/iStockphoto
9: © cyano66/iStockphoto
10: © kali9/iStockphoto
13: © AJ Watt/iStockphoto
15: © SDI Productions/iStockphoto
17: © Fred Froese/iStockphoto
19: © AnnaStills/iStockphoto
23: © Edwin Tan/iStockphoto
27: © Deagreez/iStockphoto
29: © Red Line Editorial
32: © SDI Productions/iStockphoto
35: © Obradovic/iStockphoto
37: © Phynart Studio/iStockphoto
39: © RossHelen/iStockphoto
41: © Narin Phapnam/Shutterstock Images
42: © ProfessionalStudioImages/iStockphoto
45: © Prathan Chorruangsak/iStockphoto
46: © kazuma seki/iStockphoto
49: © RealPeopleGroup/iStockphoto
51: © Zinkevych/iStockphoto
53: © RealPeopleGroup/iStockphoto
55: © xavierarnau/iStockphoto
57: © omphoto/Shutterstock Images
61: © sturti/iStockphoto
63: © CasarsaGuru/iStockphoto
65: © Geber86/iStockphoto
69: © visualspace/iStockphoto
71: © FG Trade/iStockphoto
73: © wsfurlan/iStockphoto

ABOUT THE AUTHOR

Philip Wolny is a writer and editor and a recent transplant to Florida. The large presence of seniors in his community and state, which serves as one of the nation's largest retirement destinations, has underscored to him the importance and contribution of health aides.